Table of Contents.

INTRODUCTION

The Importance of a Healthy Relationship with Food

Food is not just fuel for the body; it is a fundamental aspect of human existence that goes far beyond mere sustenance. Our relationship with food is intricate, multifaceted, and deeply intertwined with our physical, emotional, and social well-being. It is a relationship that can profoundly impact our health, happiness, and overall quality of life. At its core, a healthy relationship with food involves a balanced and harmonious approach to eating. It's about nourishing the body, mind, and soul while respecting the body's cues and signals. Such a relationship transcends diet fads, trends, and quick fixes. Instead, it fosters a sustainable and long-term connection with the food we consume. One of the key aspects of a healthy relationship with food is mindfulness. Mindful eating is the practice of being fully present and aware during meals. It involves savoring each bite, paying attention to taste and texture, and listening to the body's hunger and fullness cues. Mindful eating encourages us to eat with intention, to savor the flavors, and to appreciate the nourishment food provides. In our fast-paced modern world, the importance of slowing down and savoring our meals cannot be overstated. When we eat mindlessly—while distracted by screens, work, or other activities—we miss out on the sensory pleasure of eating. This can lead to overconsumption and dissatisfaction, as our bodies and minds crave more than what we actually need. A healthy relationship with food also means embracing variety and balance in our diet. It involves choosing a wide range of foods that provide essential nutrients, vitamins, and minerals. A varied diet not only promotes better health but also keeps our taste buds engaged and satisfied. It prevents the monotony that often leads to unhealthy cravings and binges. Furthermore, a balanced approach to food recognizes that no food is inherently "good" or "bad." It rejects the idea of labeling certain foods as forbidden or sinful. Instead, it encourages moderation and flexibility. Allowing yourself to enjoy occasional treats without guilt is an integral part of a healthy relationship with food. This moderation helps avoid the feelings of deprivation that can lead to unhealthy binge-eating behaviors. Another crucial aspect of our relationship with food is the connection between what we eat and how we feel. The food we consume has a direct impact on our physical and emotional well-being. Nutrient-dense foods, such as fruits, vegetables, whole grains, and lean proteins, provide the body with the energy and nourishment it needs to function optimally. They promote stable energy levels, enhance mental clarity, and support emotional stability. On the flip side, a diet high in processed foods, sugary drinks, and excessive amounts of unhealthy fats can lead to weight gain, chronic health conditions, and emotional instability. It can contribute to mood swings, fatigue, and increased stress levels. Therefore, our food choices not only affect our physical health but also have a profound influence on our emotional state and mental health. A healthy relationship with food acknowledges the emotional connection we have with what we eat. Food is often associated with comfort, celebration, and social gatherings. It can evoke memories, trigger cravings, and serve as a source of pleasure. However, when food becomes the primary means of coping with stress, sadness, or other emotions, it can lead to emotional eating patterns that are detrimental to our health. Recognizing and addressing emotional eating is a vital step in cultivating a healthy relationship with food. It involves finding alternative ways to manage emotions, such as practicing mindfulness, engaging in physical activity, or seeking support from friends and professionals. In addition to personal well-being, our relationship with food extends to our impact on the environment. Sustainable eating, which is becoming increasingly important in our era of climate change and resource depletion, emphasizes choosing foods that have a lower environmental footprint. This means opting for locally sourced, seasonal, and plant-based foods, as well as reducing food waste. A healthy relationship with food is not a one-size-fits-all concept but rather a holistic and individualized approach to eating. It encompasses mindfulness, variety, balance, and emotional awareness. It is about nourishing our bodies, supporting our mental and emotional health, and considering the broader impact of our food choices. By fostering a healthy relationship with food, we can enhance our overall well-being, find joy in eating, and maintain a sustainable and fulfilling connection with the nourishment that sustains us.

The Connection Between Food and Well-Being

Food is not merely sustenance; it is a fundamental aspect of human existence, intricately linked to our overall well-being. The connection between food and well-being is profound, multifaceted, and deeply rooted in both our physical and emotional lives. It encompasses not only the nourishment of our bodies but also the impact of our dietary choices on our mental and emotional health. From the earliest days of human civilization, food has played a central role in our lives. It has been a means of survival, a source of cultural identity, and a symbol of hospitality and community. The act of sharing meals has fostered bonds among individuals and societies throughout history. However, in today's fast-paced and convenience-driven world, the significance of food and its role in our well-being has sometimes been overshadowed by quick fixes and processed alternatives. At its core, food provides the essential nutrients and energy our bodies need to function. It is the fuel that powers our daily activities, from the most basic bodily functions like breathing and digestion to more complex tasks such as problem-solving and creative expression. The food we consume directly impacts our physical health, influencing factors like weight, cardiovascular health, and the risk of chronic diseases. A diet rich in whole foods—such as fruits, vegetables, whole grains, lean proteins, and healthy fats—provides the body with the necessary nutrients to thrive. These foods offer a broad spectrum of vitamins, minerals, and antioxidants that support immune function, promote cellular repair, and help maintain healthy organ systems. Conversely, a diet high in processed foods, sugars, and unhealthy fats can lead to nutritional deficiencies, obesity, and a range of health issues. The impact of food on our physical well-being is perhaps most evident in the rise of diet-related health conditions. Conditions like obesity, type 2 diabetes, cardiovascular disease, and certain cancers are closely linked to dietary choices. The prevalence of these conditions has reached epidemic proportions in many parts of the world, underscoring the importance of making informed and health-conscious decisions about what we eat. However, the connection between food and well-being extends beyond the physical realm. Increasingly, research highlights the significant influence of diet on mental and emotional health. The gut-brain connection, for instance, has gained attention as scientists uncover the intricate relationship between the digestive system and the brain.

The gut microbiome, a complex community of microorganisms living in our digestive tract, plays a crucial role in this connection. These microbes are involved in the production of neurotransmitters and other signaling molecules that affect mood and behavior. Consequently, an imbalanced gut microbiome can contribute to mood disorders like depression and anxiety. Furthermore, the foods we consume can have a direct impact on brain function and mental health. Nutrient-dense foods supply the brain with essential vitamins and minerals needed for cognitive function, memory, and emotional regulation. Omega-3 fatty acids, found in fatty fish like salmon and walnuts, have been associated with improved mood and cognitive performance.

On the flip side, a diet high in processed foods, refined sugars, and trans fats has been linked to an increased risk of depression and anxiety. These foods can lead to inflammation in the body, which, in turn, can affect brain function and contribute to mood disorders. Moreover, the act of eating itself can have profound effects on our emotional well-being. Meals are not just about sustenance; they are opportunities for connection, celebration, and relaxation. Sharing a meal with loved ones can foster a sense of belonging and social cohesion. Preparing and savoring food can be a source of pleasure, creativity, and mindfulness. Conversely, disordered eating patterns and unhealthy relationships with food can have detrimental effects on mental and emotional health. Conditions such as binge eating disorder, anorexia nervosa, and bulimia nervosa not only harm the body but also disrupt emotional equilibrium. They are often rooted in complex psychological factors and may require professional intervention. In addition to individual well-being, the connection between food and well-being extends to the broader societal and environmental context. The food choices we make have far-reaching implications for the planet. The industrialization of agriculture, overfishing, and deforestation to create space for livestock farming are contributing to environmental degradation and climate change. Sustainable eating practices, such as choosing locally sourced, seasonal, and plant-based foods, can reduce our ecological footprint and promote environmental well-being. Moreover, reducing food waste, which accounts for a significant portion of global greenhouse gas emissions, is an essential aspect of responsible and sustainable food consumption.

The connection between food and well-being is intricate and multifaceted. It encompasses the nourishment of our bodies, the impact of dietary choices on physical health, the influence of food on mental and emotional well-being, and the broader implications for society and the environment. Recognizing and nurturing this connection is essential for achieving a state of holistic well-being that encompasses both our personal health and the health of the planet. By

making informed and health-conscious choices about the food we eat, we can cultivate a deeper understanding of the profound relationship between food and well-being and pave the way for a healthier and more sustainable future.

Chapter 1. Understanding Food

The Basics Of Nutrition

Nutrition, the bedrock of our well-being, is a multidisciplinary field that spans biology, chemistry, physiology, and psychology. It encompasses the science behind how the food we consume interacts with our bodies to provide the essential elements crucial for growth, energy, and maintaining bodily functions. Our exploration of the basics of nutrition will take us through the core principles that underlie this vital area of study. At its core, nutrition revolves around understanding how the nutrients in our diet are metabolized and used by our bodies to support life. It delves into the intricate relationship between dietary choices and our health, from the prevention of diseases to the overall promotion of well-being.

The Role of Macronutrients and Micronutrients

Macronutrients, the primary classes of nutrients, constitute the foundation of our diet, providing us with energy and making up a substantial portion of our daily food intake. Carbohydrates, the primary source of energy for our bodies, consist of carbon, hydrogen, and oxygen atoms. These compounds are found in various foods, including grains, fruits, vegetables, legumes, and dairy products. Carbohydrates can be categorized as simple (sugars) or complex (starches and fibers). When we consume carbohydrates, they are broken down into glucose, a sugar that serves as the body's immediate energy source or is stored as glycogen in the liver and muscles for future use. Proteins are integral to the growth, repair, and maintenance of our body tissues. Comprised of amino acids, the building blocks of proteins, they are sourced from a variety of foods, including animal products such as meat, poultry, fish, and dairy, as well as plant-based sources like legumes, nuts, and seeds. While some amino acids can be synthesized by the body, others are considered essential amino acids and must be obtained through our diet. Dietary fats are a concentrated source of energy and play a vital role in absorbing fat-soluble vitamins (A, D, E, and K). They are composed of fatty acids and glycerol. Fats can be saturated (found in animal products and some plant oils) or unsaturated (found in plant oils, fatty fish, and nuts). Unsaturated fats, including monounsaturated and polyunsaturated fats, are considered healthier for heart health and overall well-being.

Micronutrients encompass vitamins and minerals, which our bodies require in smaller quantities but are vital for various physiological processes. Vitamins, organic compounds, act as regulators of bodily functions. They fall into two categories: water-soluble vitamins (e.g., vitamin C and B vitamins) and fat-soluble vitamins (e.g., vitamins A, D, E, and K). Each vitamin has specific roles in maintaining health, such as supporting the immune system (vitamin C), promoting bone health (vitamin D), and acting as antioxidants (vitamin E). Minerals, inorganic nutrients, are crucial for various bodily functions. Essential minerals include calcium (important for bone health), iron (critical for oxygen transport), magnesium (essential for muscle and nerve function), and potassium (necessary for maintaining fluid balance). Trace minerals like zinc and selenium are needed in smaller quantities but are still vital for health.

Water, often overlooked as a nutrient, is the most vital one. It constitutes a substantial portion of our body weight and is involved in nearly every physiological process, from digestion and circulation to temperature regulation and waste removal. Staying adequately hydrated is essential for overall health and well-being.

The nutritional journey begins with the digestion and absorption of nutrients from the foods we consume. Digestion is the process by which food is broken down into smaller, more manageable components. It begins in the mouth, where enzymes in saliva initiate the breakdown of carbohydrates. In the stomach, gastric juices break down proteins, and in the small intestine, digestive enzymes further break down carbohydrates, proteins, and fats. After digestion, nutrients are absorbed through the walls of the small intestine and transported to various cells and tissues in the body via the bloodstream. Nutrients such as glucose (from carbohydrates), amino acids (from proteins), and fatty acids (from fats) are absorbed into the bloodstream and used for energy, growth, and repair.

Balancing energy intake (calories consumed through food) with energy expenditure (calories burned through physical activity and metabolic processes) is pivotal for maintaining a healthy weight. When energy intake exceeds expenditure, excess calories are stored as fat, leading to weight gain. Conversely, if energy expenditure surpasses intake, the body taps into stored energy (fat) for fuel, resulting in weight loss.

Nutritional guidelines offer recommendations on dietary patterns that promote health and reduce the risk of chronic diseases. They emphasize:
- A balanced diet, comprising a variety of foods from all food groups to ensure the body receives all essential nutrients in appropriate amounts.
- Portion control, preventing overconsumption of calories and promoting weight management.
- Limiting sugars and saturated fats, reducing the risk of obesity, heart disease, and other health issues.
- Eating whole foods, such as fruits, vegetables, whole grains, and lean proteins, is associated with better health outcomes.
- Staying adequately hydrated is essential for overall health, as water supports numerous bodily functions.
Individual dietary needs can vary based on factors such as age, gender, activity level, and underlying health conditions. Special diets, such as vegetarianism, veganism, gluten-free diets, and low-carb diets, may be adopted for various reasons. Tailoring dietary choices to individual needs and consulting healthcare professionals when necessary is vital.
Nutrition serves as the cornerstone of human health and well-being. The foods we consume provide the essential macronutrients, micronutrients, and water required for the body to function optimally. Understanding the basics of nutrition empowers individuals to make informed dietary choices, support their physical and mental health, and reduce the risk of chronic diseases. Embracing a balanced and mindful approach to nutrition allows individuals to cultivate a lifelong commitment to health and well-being.

Food Groups and Their Importance

Food is the sustenance of life, and the choices we make regarding what we eat have profound implications for our health and well-

being. To understand the significance of these choices, we need to examine the concept of food groups, which categorizes foods based on their nutrient content and helps us make informed dietary decisions. Food groups provide a framework for balanced eating by ensuring that we get a variety of essential nutrients from our diets. Understanding the significance of these groups is crucial for maintaining good health and preventing nutrition-related diseases. Let's delve into the major food groups and explore their importance in our daily lives. Grains are one of the fundamental food groups and serve as a primary source of carbohydrates, which are the body's main source of energy. This group includes foods made from wheat, rice, oats, corn, barley, and other grains. Some common grain products include bread, pasta, cereal, and rice. The importance of grains lies in their role as an energy provider. Carbohydrates in grains are converted into glucose, which our bodies use for energy. Grains also provide essential vitamins and minerals, such as B vitamins (e.g., thiamine, riboflavin, niacin), iron, and dietary fiber. Whole grains, such as whole wheat bread and brown rice, offer additional benefits because they retain the bran and germ layers of the grain, which contain fiber, vitamins, and minerals. Fiber aids in digestion, helps maintain stable blood sugar levels, and supports heart health. Vegetables are a rich source of vitamins, minerals, fiber, and antioxidants. This food group includes a wide variety of plant-based foods, such as leafy greens, root vegetables, legumes, and cruciferous vegetables like broccoli and cauliflower. The importance of vegetables in our diets cannot be overstated. They are a powerhouse of essential nutrients, including vitamins A, C, and K, as well as folate, potassium, and dietary fiber. These nutrients play vital roles in maintaining healthy skin, vision, immune function, and digestion. Consuming a diverse range of vegetables is key to reaping their full benefits. Different vegetables provide different nutrients, so incorporating a variety into your diet ensures a broader spectrum of health benefits.

Fruits, like vegetables, are rich in vitamins, minerals, antioxidants, and dietary fiber. This food group encompasses a wide array of naturally sweet and colorful foods, such as apples, bananas, oranges, berries, and citrus fruits. The importance of fruits lies in their contribution to overall health and well-being. They are particularly known for being excellent sources of vitamin C, potassium, and dietary fiber. Vitamin C is crucial for skin health

and immune function, while potassium helps regulate blood pressure and muscle function. The natural sugars in fruits provide a healthier alternative to added sugars found in processed foods and sugary beverages. Incorporating a variety of fruits into your diet can satisfy your sweet tooth while providing essential nutrients. Proteins are essential for building and repairing tissues, producing enzymes and hormones, and supporting overall growth and development. This food group includes a wide range of sources, such as meat, poultry, fish, eggs, dairy products, legumes, and nuts. The importance of protein in our diets cannot be overstated. Proteins are composed of amino acids, which are the building blocks of the body. Some amino acids are produced by the body, while others must be obtained through the diet. These essential amino acids are found in various protein sources, making it important to consume a variety of proteins to ensure adequate intake. Lean protein sources, such as poultry, fish, beans, and tofu, provide the necessary protein without excessive saturated fats, making them heart-healthy choices. Additionally, seafood is a valuable source of omega-3 fatty acids, which have been linked to various health benefits, including heart health and brain function.

Dairy products are rich in calcium and other essential nutrients like vitamin D, potassium, and protein. This food group includes milk, yogurt, cheese, and fortified plant-based alternatives like almond or soy milk. The importance of dairy lies in its role in bone health. Calcium is essential for building and maintaining strong bones and teeth, and vitamin D aids in calcium absorption. Dairy products are among the best dietary sources of calcium, making them a critical component of bone health, especially in growing children and older adults. For those who are lactose intolerant or prefer plant-based options, fortified plant-based milk alternatives can provide similar nutrients. Look for products that are fortified with calcium and vitamin D to ensure you're getting the same benefits as traditional dairy.

Fats and oils are concentrated sources of energy and provide essential fatty acids, such as omega-3 and omega-6 fatty acids.

This food group includes sources like oils (olive oil, canola oil), nuts, seeds, avocados, and fatty fish (salmon, mackerel).
The importance of fats and oils lies in their role as an energy source and in supporting overall health. Dietary fats are necessary for absorbing fat-soluble vitamins (A, D, E, and K), protecting

organs, and regulating body temperature. Additionally, omega-3 fatty acids, found in fatty fish, are associated with reduced inflammation, improved heart health, and cognitive benefits. It's crucial to choose healthy fats, such as monounsaturated and polyunsaturated fats found in olive oil, nuts, and fatty fish, over saturated and trans fats found in processed and fried foods. A balanced intake of fats and oils contributes to overall well-being and cardiovascular health. The sweets and sugars group includes foods and beverages high in added sugars, such as candy, soft drinks, and desserts. While these items may add flavor and enjoyment to our diets, they should be consumed in moderation due to their low nutritional value and potential negative health effects. The importance of managing sweets and sugars lies in their impact on overall health. Consuming excessive added sugars is associated with various health issues, including obesity, type 2 diabetes, heart disease, and dental problems. Reducing sugar intake and choosing whole foods and fruits as sweet alternatives can help maintain a balanced diet and support health. Water is a crucial nutrient often overlooked in food group discussions. It is essential for life and plays a foundational role in various bodily functions. While water isn't classified as a traditional food group, it deserves special attention due to its significance. The importance of water cannot be overstated. It makes up a significant portion of our body weight and is involved in nearly every physiological process, including digestion, circulation, temperature regulation, and waste removal. Staying adequately hydrated is essential for overall health and well-being. Balanced eating is about incorporating foods from all food groups into your diet to ensure you receive a wide array of essential nutrients. A balanced diet supports overall health, provides energy, and reduces the risk of nutrition-related diseases. Dietary guidelines, such as those provided by government health agencies, offer recommendations on dietary patterns that promote health and well-being.

These guidelines typically emphasize:
- Balancing food groups: Including foods from all food groups to ensure a diverse intake of nutrients.
- Portion control: Managing portion sizes to prevent overconsumption of calories and support weight management.

- Limiting added sugars and unhealthy fats: Reducing the intake of added sugars and saturated and trans fats to lower the risk of chronic diseases.
- Eating whole foods: Incorporating whole foods, such Nutrition, the bedrock of our well-being, is a multidisciplinary field that spans biology, chemistry, physiology, and psychology. It encompasses the science behind how the food we consume interacts with our bodies to provide the essential elements crucial for growth, energy, and maintaining bodily functions. Our exploration of the basics of nutrition will take us through the core principles that underlie this vital area of study. At its core, nutrition revolves around understanding how the nutrients in our diet are metabolized and used by our bodies to support life. It delves into the intricate relationship between dietary choices and our health, from the prevention of diseases to the overall promotion of well-being.

Chapter 2.
Mindful Eating

The Power of Mindful Eating

In a fast-paced world where meals are often consumed in haste or skipped altogether, the concept of mindful eating emerges as a beacon of awareness and nourishment. Mindful eating is not merely a diet or a quick fix; it is a profound shift in the way we relate to food, our bodies, and the world around us. At its core, mindful eating is about being fully present in the act of eating, fostering a deeper connection with the food we consume, and understanding the intricate interplay between mind, body, and sustenance. In this exploration of the power of mindful eating, we will delve into its benefits, practical steps to practice it, and the transformative impact it can have on our lives.

The Benefits of Mindful Eating
Mindful eating is not just a passing trend but a practice deeply rooted in ancient wisdom and backed by modern science. Its benefits extend far beyond the plate, touching various aspects of our physical, emotional, and mental well-being. The profound effects of mindful eating unfold in a holistic manner, offering a new perspective on our relationship with food and ourselves.

First and foremost, mindful eating encourages a heightened sense of awareness. It invites us to engage all our senses when approaching a meal—the sight, smell, texture, and taste of the food come alive in a way that transcends mere consumption. This heightened awareness leads to a deeper appreciation for the culinary experience, turning each meal into a sensory delight rather than a rushed necessity. Moreover, mindful eating promotes a healthier relationship with food. It frees us from the shackles of restrictive diets, counting calories, or succumbing to mindless emotional eating. Instead, it cultivates a profound understanding of hunger and satiety cues. By listening to our bodies, we learn to eat when hungry and stop when satisfied, thus naturally regulating our portions and fostering healthier weight management. Furthermore, mindful eating has been shown to reduce overeating and binge eating tendencies. By paying close attention to the signals our body sends, we become attuned to the subtle distinctions between physical hunger and emotional cravings. This heightened awareness empowers us to make conscious choices rather than surrendering to impulsive and often unhealthy eating habits. Mindful eating is also a powerful tool for managing and preventing various health conditions. Research indicates that it can be instrumental in managing weight, improving glycemic control in individuals with diabetes, and even alleviating symptoms of irritable bowel syndrome (IBS). By fostering a deep connection with the act of eating, it enables us to make informed choices that support our health and well-being. In addition to its physical benefits, mindful eating has a profound impact on our emotional and psychological well-being. It is a practice rooted in self-compassion, encouraging us to approach ourselves and our eating habits with kindness and non-judgment. This self-compassion extends beyond the dining table, promoting a positive body image and reducing the prevalence of disordered eating behaviors.

Mindful eating is a powerful stress management tool. In a world where stress often leads to mindless snacking and emotional eating, it offers a respite. By bringing our full attention to the present moment and the act of eating, we create a buffer against the stresses of life. This practice enables us to respond to stressors with greater resilience and equanimity, reducing the reliance on comfort foods as a coping mechanism. Mindful eating has the potential to enhance our overall mental well-being. It encourages a meditative approach to eating, fostering a sense of calm and tranquility. This state of mindfulness not only transforms our relationship with food but also has a ripple effect on our mental state. It has been associated with reduced symptoms of anxiety and depression, providing a holistic approach to emotional wellness.

Practical Steps to Practice Mindful Eating

Practicing mindful eating is not a complex endeavor; it is accessible to anyone willing to cultivate a more mindful approach to their meals. It is a skill that can be honed with patience and practice, gradually transforming the way we engage with food. Here are practical steps to embark on a journey toward mindful eating:

Begin with Awareness

To truly practice mindful eating, it all begins with awareness. This foundational step is the cornerstone of the mindful eating journey. Awareness invites us to be fully present in the moment, to engage our senses, and to pay undivided attention to the act of eating. It means slowing down the pace of our meals, setting aside distractions like phones or television, and creating a sacred space for our culinary experience. Starting with awareness involves observing our thoughts, emotions, and bodily sensations before, during, and after meals. It's about tuning into our hunger and fullness cues, which are the body's natural signals that guide our eating. Are we eating because we are genuinely hungry, or are external factors like stress, boredom, or social pressure influencing our choices? By being acutely aware of our motives, we can make conscious decisions about when, what, and how much to eat. Moreover, awareness extends to the food itself. We can take the time to truly look at our meal, appreciate its colors, textures, and presentation. We can savor the aroma, inhaling deeply to fully engage our sense of smell. As we take that first bite, we experience the explosion of flavors on our taste buds, noting the subtleties and nuances of each ingredient. By immersing ourselves in this sensory experience, we cultivate a deeper connection with our food. Beginning with awareness also involves non-judgmental observation. We refrain from labeling foods as "good" or "bad" and relinquish the guilt or shame often associated with eating. Instead, we approach our meals with curiosity and compassion. If we find ourselves indulging in a treat or an occasional indulgence, we acknowledge it without criticism, recognizing that moderation and balance are key principles of mindful eating. Furthermore, awareness encompasses the recognition of our eating habits and patterns. Do we tend to rush through meals, barely tasting our food? Are we prone to emotional eating, seeking comfort in snacks when stressed or sad? By observing these habits without judgment, we gain insight into our behavior and pave the way for positive change. In essence, beginning with awareness in the practice of mindful eating is about creating a space for presence and connection with ourselves and our food. It allows us to make deliberate choices that align with our physical and emotional needs, ultimately fostering a healthier and more fulfilling relationship with eating. By cultivating this awareness at each meal, we embark on a transformative journey toward greater well-being and a profound appreciation for the nourishment that food can provide.

Savor Each Bite

Savoring each bite is a central and transformative aspect of mindful eating. It involves bringing our full attention to the eating experience, immersing ourselves in the sensory pleasure of each mouthful. This practice encourages us to slow down, to appreciate the textures, flavors, and aromas of our food, and to engage all our senses in the act of eating. When we savor each bite, we create a profound connection with our food. We take the time to look at our meal, admiring its colors and presentation. We savor the smell of the dish, allowing the aroma to tantalize our senses. As we take that first bite, we experience a symphony of flavors on our taste buds, from sweet and savory to bitter and umami. Savoring involves paying attention to the way the food feels in our mouths, its temperature, and the sound of our chewing. This heightened awareness of the eating experience not only enhances our enjoyment of food but also promotes mindfulness. By savoring each bite, we stay fully present in the moment, preventing mindless eating, where we consume food almost mechanically without truly tasting or appreciating it. Savoring slows the pace of our meals, allowing our bodies to recognize feelings of fullness, which can help prevent overeating. Furthermore, savoring promotes a sense of gratitude for the nourishment we receive from our food. It encourages us to acknowledge the effort and care that may have gone into preparing the meal, whether by ourselves or others. This gratitude can deepen our connection with food and foster a positive relationship with eating, free from guilt or shame.

Savoring each bite can be a gateway to exploring new flavors and cuisines. It encourages culinary curiosity and the willingness to try foods that may be unfamiliar. By savoring different tastes and textures, we expand our palate and open ourselves to a world of culinary delights. Savoring each bite is a practice that not only enhances the enjoyment of our meals but also cultivates mindfulness, gratitude, and a deeper connection with food. It encourages us to slow down, engage our senses, and savor the full experience of eating. By incorporating this practice into our daily lives, we embark on a journey toward greater well-being and a more profound appreciation for the nourishing and pleasurable aspects of food.

Listen to Your Body
Listening to your body is a fundamental and transformative aspect of practicing mindful eating. It involves tuning in to the signals and cues your body provides, both physical and emotional, to guide your eating choices. This practice encourages you to trust your body's innate wisdom and respond to its needs with compassion and understanding. When you listen to your body, you become attuned to hunger and fullness cues. You learn to distinguish between true physical hunger and other impulses to eat, such as emotional or social triggers. By paying attention to your body's signals of hunger, you can eat when you genuinely need nourishment and stop when you're satisfied, preventing overeating or mindless consumption. Moreover, this practice fosters a deeper connection with your body's unique needs and preferences. It acknowledges that no one-size-fits-all approach to eating exists and that your body's requirements may vary from day to day. By listening to your body, you become more responsive to its cravings, dietary preferences, and sensitivities. You honor your body's signals for specific nutrients, helping you make informed choices that align with your well-being. Listening to your body also involves recognizing emotional cues related to eating. It encourages you to pause and reflect on the underlying emotions that may influence your food choices. Are you eating out of stress, boredom, sadness, or genuine hunger? By acknowledging these emotions without judgment, you can develop healthier coping mechanisms and address emotional eating with mindfulness and self-compassion. This practice further promotes flexibility in your eating patterns. It encourages you to be adaptable and responsive to your body's needs, allowing you to enjoy a wide range of foods and culinary experiences without rigid dietary rules or restrictions. It invites you to savor food without guilt and to indulge occasionally without judgment. Listening to your body is also about respecting your body's boundaries and limitations. It means recognizing when you've had enough and respecting your body's need for rest and nourishment. It discourages pushing yourself to eat or restrict food based on external pressures, societal expectations, or dieting rules.

Listening to your body is a practice that honors the wisdom and needs of your body. It involves tuning in to hunger and fullness cues, recognizing emotional triggers, and respecting your body's unique requirements and preferences. By incorporating this practice into your daily life, you embark on a journey toward greater self-awareness, a healthier relationship with food, and a profound connection with your body's innate wisdom and well-being.

Mindful Portion Control

Mindful portion control is an essential element of practicing mindful eating. It involves being conscious of the quantity of food you consume while paying close attention to your body's hunger and fullness cues. This practice empowers you to enjoy your meals in a balanced and nourishing way, preventing overeating and promoting a healthier relationship with food. One key aspect of mindful portion control is serving yourself with intention. Rather than piling your plate mindlessly or adhering to external portion sizes, you take a moment to assess your hunger and choose an appropriate amount of food. This practice allows you to honor your body's needs and helps prevent the habit of eating beyond fullness. Mindful portion control also encourages you to savor each bite and eat slowly. By slowing down the pace of your meals, you give your body the time it needs to register feelings of fullness, which can prevent overconsumption. It allows you to enjoy the sensory experience of eating and promotes mindfulness throughout the meal. Another crucial aspect is paying attention to portion sizes in different contexts, such as dining out or when faced with larger servings. Mindful portion control equips you with strategies to navigate these situations with confidence and moderation. It encourages you to listen to your body's cues, even when external portions may be larger than what you need. This practice helps you develop an awareness of portion distortion, a common phenomenon where external cues influence your perception of how much you should eat. By recognizing this distortion and making choices based on your actual hunger, you can maintain a healthier relationship with food and portion sizes. Furthermore, mindful portion control emphasizes the quality of the food you choose rather than just the quantity. It encourages you to select nutrient-dense foods that provide essential nutrients and satisfaction in smaller quantities. This approach allows you to enjoy the flavors and benefits of your meal without needing to consume excessive amounts.Mindful portion control is about making conscious choices regarding the amount of food you eat, based on your body's cues and your intention to nourish yourself effectively. It emphasizes serving with intention, savoring each bite, and being mindful of portion sizes in various contexts. By incorporating this practice into your daily eating habits, you can foster a balanced and positive relationship with food, ultimately supporting your well-being and satisfaction with meals.

Engage Your Senses

Engaging your senses is a pivotal aspect of the mindful eating practice, infusing each meal with a deeper and more meaningful connection to your food. This approach encourages you to fully immerse yourself in the sensory experience of eating, creating a heightened awareness of the flavors, textures, aromas, and visual appeal of your meal. One of the primary senses engaged in mindful eating is taste. By savoring each bite, you allow the rich tapestry of flavors to dance on your taste buds. You notice the subtle nuances of sweet, sour, salty, bitter, and umami, appreciating the intricate balance of ingredients that contribute to the overall taste of your food. This sensory engagement elevates your eating experience, making it more pleasurable and satisfying. Engaging your sense of smell is equally crucial in mindful eating. The aroma of food can be captivating, triggering memories and evoking emotions. Taking a moment to inhale deeply and savor the scents of your meal enhances the overall sensory experience, intensifying your connection to the food and increasing your mindfulness. Engaging your sense of touch involves paying attention to the textures and temperatures of your food. You notice the contrast between crispy and soft, hot and cold, smooth and rough. This sensory awareness adds depth to your eating experience, allowing you to appreciate the diversity of sensations that food provides.

Visual appeal is another vital component of engaging your senses. The presentation of a meal, the colors on your plate, and the visual harmony of ingredients all contribute to your sensory experience. By taking a moment to admire your food, you not only enhance your enjoyment but also cultivate mindfulness, making each meal a more conscious and intentional act. Engaging your senses in mindful eating fosters a profound connection to your food and the present moment. It encourages you to slow down, savor each bite, and fully appreciate the nourishment and pleasure that food brings. This practice promotes a greater awareness of your body's hunger and fullness cues, preventing overeating and helping you make healthier choices. By incorporating this sensory mindfulness into your eating habits, you enrich your relationship with food, making each meal a delightful and nourishing experience.

Slow Down

Slowing down is a fundamental and transformative component of practicing mindful eating. In a fast-paced world where rushed meals and hectic schedules have become the norm, this practice invites us to pause and savor the present moment. It encourages us to eat at a more deliberate and mindful pace, fostering a deeper connection with our food and our bodies. When we slow down, we allow ourselves the time to fully engage with the sensory experience of eating. Each bite becomes an opportunity to appreciate the flavors, textures, and aromas of our meal. We become more attuned to the subtleties of taste, distinguishing between sweet, salty, sour, bitter, and umami flavors, and savoring the intricate interplay of ingredients. This heightened sensory awareness transforms our meals into moments of pleasure and satisfaction. Slowing down also extends to the act of chewing and swallowing. Mindful eating encourages us to chew our food thoroughly, savoring each bite before proceeding to the next. This deliberate chewing not only enhances our enjoyment but also aids in digestion, as it allows our bodies to break down food more effectively. By being present with each mouthful, we reduce the likelihood of overeating and become more attuned to our body's signals of fullness. Slowing down promotes mindfulness throughout the meal. It discourages mindless eating, where we consume food rapidly without truly savoring or appreciating it. By eating slowly and consciously, we become more aware of our body's hunger cues, helping us make better choices about when and how much to eat. Slowing down also allows us to reconnect with the social and cultural aspects of eating. Meals become an opportunity to engage in conversation, share stories, and strengthen our relationships with family and friends. This practice fosters a sense of togetherness and community, reminding us that food is not only about nourishment but also about connection and enjoyment. Slowing down is an essential practice in mindful eating that invites us to fully engage with our meals and the present moment. It enhances our sensory awareness, promotes mindful chewing and swallowing, and encourages a more deliberate and conscious approach to eating. By incorporating this practice into our daily lives, we not only enrich our relationship with food but also nourish our bodies, minds, and spirits with the mindfulness and presence that it brings.

Practice Gratitude

Practicing gratitude within the context of mindful eating can transform your relationship with food into a deeply enriching experience. This practice encourages you to cultivate an attitude of appreciation and thankfulness for the nourishment that food provides. It is a simple yet profound act that can bring a sense of joy, contentment, and mindfulness to your meals. When you practice gratitude, you take a moment before eating to acknowledge the journey that your food has taken from its source to your plate. You appreciate the effort that may have gone into growing, harvesting, preparing, and transporting the ingredients. This awareness not only fosters a greater connection with your food but also instills a sense of reverence for the Earth and the people who contribute to your meal. Moreover, gratitude encourages you to be fully present with your food, savoring each bite with a sense of appreciation. It shifts your focus away from mere consumption and toward a deeper understanding of the nourishment and sustenance that food provides. This shift in perspective allows you to approach your meals with a sense of abundance and mindfulness, reducing the tendency to overeat or eat mindlessly. Practicing gratitude can also promote a positive and joyful relationship with food. It encourages you to let go of any guilt or shame associated with eating and to embrace a more compassionate and accepting attitude towards your dietary choices. By recognizing the value of nourishing your body and soul, you create a harmonious and balanced approach to eating that extends far beyond the plate. Gratitude reminds you to be thankful for your own body and its ability to process and utilize the nutrients from your food. It encourages you to treat your body with kindness and care, choosing foods that support your overall well-being. This act of self-appreciation can lead to more conscious and nourishing food choices. practicing gratitude in the context of mindful eating is a transformative practice that enriches your relationship with food. It encourages you to appreciate the journey of your food, be present with each bite, reduce overeating, and foster a positive and joyful attitude towards eating. By incorporating this practice into your meals, you not only nourish your body but also nurture a deep sense of gratitude and mindfulness that can enhance your overall well-being.

Minimize Distractions

Minimizing distractions is a cornerstone of mindful eating, allowing you to create a sacred space for your meals and fully engage in the experience. In a world filled with constant stimuli, it's all too easy to consume food mindlessly while multitasking or being absorbed in digital devices. The practice of minimizing distractions encourages you to bring your complete attention to the act of eating, fostering a deeper connection with your food and your body. By removing distractions such as television, smartphones, or work-related tasks during mealtime, you create an environment that promotes mindfulness. This intentional focus on eating enables you to savor the flavors, textures, and aromas of your food, enhancing the sensory experience. It also allows you to pay attention to your body's hunger and fullness cues, helping you make informed choices about when to start and stop eating. Minimizing distractions during meals also promotes mindful chewing and swallowing. It encourages you to take the time to thoroughly chew your food, aiding in digestion and ensuring that you receive the full nutritional benefit from your meal. This practice can prevent mindless overeating, as you become more attuned to your body's signals of fullness. Minimizing distractions fosters a sense of presence and connection with the people you may be sharing your meal with. It encourages meaningful conversations and strengthens your relationships by allowing you to engage fully in the social aspect of dining. This practice reinforces the idea that mealtime is not just about nourishing the body but also about nurturing connections and fostering a sense of togetherness. It is also a fundamental practice in mindful eating that encourages you to create a mindful and intentional eating environment. It enables you to fully engage with your food, heighten sensory awareness, and listen to your body's cues. By incorporating this practice into your meals, you can embrace a more mindful and fulfilling relationship with food while deepening your connections with others.

Cultivate Mindful Snacking

Cultivating mindful snacking is an integral aspect of practicing mindful eating that extends beyond your main meals. This practice encourages you to approach snacks with the same mindfulness and intention as your regular meals, fostering a balanced and nourishing relationship with food throughout the day. Mindful snacking begins with awareness of your body's hunger cues. It invites you to check in with yourself and determine whether you're truly hungry or experiencing a non-physical trigger for eating, such as stress or boredom. By being attuned to your body's signals, you can make conscious decisions about when to snack and when to honor your hunger. Moreover, mindful snacking encourages you to select snacks that align with your nutritional needs and preferences. It emphasizes choosing nutrient-dense options that provide sustenance and satisfaction rather than empty calories. This practice allows you to make informed choices that support your overall well-being. Cultivating mindfulness during snacking also involves slowing down and savoring each bite. It discourages mindless, rapid consumption and encourages you to engage your senses fully. By taking the time to enjoy the flavors and textures of your snack, you not only enhance your sensory experience but also prevent overeating. Mindful snacking promotes a sense of gratitude for the nourishment that snacks provide. It encourages you to acknowledge the value of these smaller meals and the role they play in sustaining your energy and satiety between larger meals. This sense of appreciation can lead to a healthier and more balanced approach to snacking. Cultivating mindful snacking is an essential practice within the realm of mindful eating. It involves being aware of your body's hunger cues, selecting nutrient-dense options, savoring each bite, and fostering gratitude for the nourishment snacks offer. By incorporating this practice into your daily routine, you can develop a more conscious and balanced relationship with food, promoting overall well-being and satisfaction with your dietary choices.

Practice Mindful Drinking

Practicing mindful drinking is an often-overlooked but crucial component of mindful eating, as what we drink can significantly impact our overall well-being and relationship with food. This practice encourages you to be fully present and intentional in your choices of beverages, promoting hydration, nourishment, and sensory awareness. Mindful drinking begins with the awareness of your body's thirst cues. It invites you to tune in and recognize when you're genuinely thirsty rather than reaching for a drink out of habit or in response to non-physical triggers. By paying attention to your body's signals, you can ensure that you stay adequately hydrated, which is essential for overall health. Moreover, mindful drinking encourages you to choose beverages that align with your well-being. It emphasizes opting for options that provide hydration, nourishment, and pleasure. Water, herbal teas, and fresh juices can be excellent choices that not only quench your thirst but also offer additional health benefits. This practice discourages excessive consumption of sugary, highly processed, or calorie-laden drinks. Cultivating mindfulness during drinking also involves savoring the sensory experience of your beverage. Just as with food, mindful drinking encourages you to engage your senses fully. You can appreciate the aroma, taste, and temperature of your drink, making each sip a moment of pleasure and refreshment. This heightened sensory awareness adds depth and satisfaction to your beverage consumption. Practicing mindful drinking invites you to recognize the value of hydration in supporting your overall well-being. It encourages gratitude for the simple act of quenching your thirst and nourishing your body with essential fluids. This sense of appreciation can deepen your connection with your body's needs and reinforce the importance of mindful hydration in your daily life. Practicing mindful drinking is an integral part of mindful eating that promotes hydration, nourishment, and sensory awareness. It involves recognizing your body's thirst cues, choosing beverages that align with your well-being, savoring the sensory experience, and fostering gratitude for the simple act of staying hydrated. By incorporating this practice into your daily routine, you can enhance your relationship with beverages and support your overall well-being.

Be Patient with Yourself

Being patient with yourself is an essential and often overlooked aspect of mindful eating. In a world that often values quick fixes and instant results, practicing patience can be a transformative and empowering approach to your relationship with food. Mindful eating is not something that you can master overnight. It's a journey, a process of developing a healthier and more conscious connection with your food and your body. As with any journey, it's important to be patient with yourself and to understand that progress may come in small, incremental steps. This patience allows you to navigate the inevitable ups and downs without becoming discouraged. One of the key elements of patience in mindful eating is recognizing that it's okay to make mistakes. It's common to slip into old eating habits, to eat mindlessly, or to overindulge from time to time. Instead of berating yourself for these lapses, practicing patience involves treating yourself with kindness and compassion. It's about acknowledging that everyone has moments of imperfection and that these moments do not define your overall progress. Patience encourages you to let go of unrealistic expectations and rigid dietary rules. It's about understanding that there's no one-size-fits-all approach to mindful eating. What works for one person may not work for another, and that's perfectly okay. By allowing yourself the space to explore what works best for you, you can develop a more individualized and sustainable approach to mindful eating. Moreover, patience involves embracing the learning process. It's about being curious and open to discovering new insights about your eating habits, your body's signals, and your emotional relationship with food. It's recognizing that self-discovery and growth take time and that each step forward, no matter how small, is a valuable part of your journey. Practicing patience in mindful eating also means understanding that change can be gradual. It may take time for you to fully incorporate mindfulness into your eating habits and to see significant shifts in your relationship with food. Patience allows you to trust in the process and to focus on the journey rather than fixating on quick results. Moreover, being patient with yourself in mindful eating is about recognizing that the goal is not perfection but progress. It's about acknowledging your efforts and celebrating your successes, no matter how small they may seem. Each mindful meal, each moment of self-awareness, and each choice aligned with your well-being is a step in the right direction. Being patient with yourself is a foundational and empowering aspect of mindful eating. It's about embracing the journey of self-discovery and growth, understanding that mistakes are part of the process, and letting go of unrealistic expectations. By practicing patience, you create the space for a more compassionate and sustainable relationship with food, allowing you to navigate the path of mindful eating with resilience and self-kindness.

Reflect on Your Experience

Reflecting on your experience is a pivotal step in the practice of mindful eating, as it allows you to deepen your self-awareness, gain valuable insights, and make informed choices regarding your relationship with food. This practice encourages you to take a moment after each meal or eating experience to contemplate your thoughts, emotions, and physical sensations. One of the key aspects of reflection in mindful eating is acknowledging any emotions or thoughts that arise during the meal. Did you experience joy, guilt, stress, or pleasure while eating? Were there any specific triggers or patterns in your thinking related to your food choices? By recognizing and naming your emotions and thoughts, you can gain clarity about your emotional relationship with food, helping you make more conscious choices in the future. Reflection also involves tuning into your body's physical sensations. How did the food make you feel physically? Did you notice any signs of fullness or satisfaction? By paying attention to your body's cues, you can learn to differentiate between physical hunger and emotional cravings, enabling you to make more mindful decisions about when to eat and when to stop. Reflection encourages you to assess your level of mindfulness during the meal. Were you fully present, engaged with your food, and savoring each bite? Or did your mind wander, and were you distracted by external factors? This self-awareness can help you identify areas for improvement and develop strategies to enhance your mindfulness in future eating experiences. Additionally, reflection invites you to consider the overall context of your meal. Were you eating alone or with others? Did the environment or social dynamics influence your eating habits? By examining the context, you can gain a deeper understanding of the external factors that may impact your food choices and your relationship with eating.

Reflection is an opportunity to express gratitude for the nourishment and satisfaction that your meal provided. It encourages you to cultivate a sense of appreciation for the food, your body, and the experience of eating. This practice of gratitude can foster a more positive and fulfilling relationship with food and promote an overall sense of well-being. Reflecting on your experience is a foundational and transformative step in mindful eating. It involves acknowledging your emotions and thoughts, tuning into your body's physical sensations, assessing your level of mindfulness, considering the meal's context, and cultivating gratitude. By incorporating this practice into your eating habits, you deepen your self-awareness, gain valuable insights, and make informed choices that support a healthier and more mindful relationship with food. The power of mindful eating transcends the realm of mere nutrition; it encompasses a profound transformation in our relationship with food, our bodies, and our overall well-being. Its benefits extend beyond the plate, touching various aspects of our physical, emotional, and mental health. By practicing mindfulness in our eating habits, we embark on a journey of self-discovery, self-compassion, and holistic wellness. Mindful eating empowers us to approach each meal with intention, gratitude, and presence, enriching our lives one bite at a time.

Techniques for Mindful Eating

Mindful eating, rooted in ancient wisdom and supported by contemporary research, is a transformative approach to nourishment that invites us to be fully present in the act of eating. It transcends the hurried, distracted consumption that often characterizes our modern eating habits. Instead, it encourages us to engage all our senses, fostering a deeper connection with the food we consume and the sensations that arise as a result. In this exploration of techniques for mindful eating, we will uncover practical steps that can be seamlessly integrated into daily life, empowering us to cultivate mindfulness in our relationship with food and, by extension, our overall well-being. One fundamental technique for mindful eating is the practice of slowing down. In our fast-paced world, meals are often rushed affairs, with little attention given to the act of eating itself. Mindful eating urges us to reverse this trend, encouraging us to decelerate our eating pace.

This practice involves chewing slowly and deliberately, savoring each bite, and putting down utensils between mouthfuls. Slowing down allows us to fully experience the flavors, textures, and sensations of the food. It not only enhances the culinary experience but also provides an opportunity to recognize and respond to our body's cues of hunger and fullness.

Listening to our body is another cornerstone of mindful eating. The technique revolves around tuning in to the signals our body sends during a meal. By paying close attention to physical sensations, such as hunger pangs or a feeling of fullness, we can discern whether we are truly hungry or simply eating out of habit, boredom, or emotional triggers. This heightened awareness empowers us to make conscious choices about when and how much to eat. It aligns our eating patterns with our body's natural rhythms and helps prevent overeating, which often results from eating mindlessly or in response to emotional cues rather than genuine hunger. Mindful portion control complements the practice of listening to our body. It involves being conscious of the portion sizes we consume. Rather than relying on external cues, such as large plates or serving sizes dictated by others, mindful portion control encourages us to trust our internal cues of hunger and fullness. Smaller plates and utensils can be used to help regulate portion sizes. However, the focus is not on rigidly restricting portions but on eating until we are comfortably satisfied, not overly full. It's a practice of balance and attunement to our body's needs. Creating a mindful eating environment is a technique that supports the practice of mindfulness during meals. This involves minimizing distractions and setting the stage for a focused and intentional eating experience. To create such an environment, we can turn off the television, put away our smartphones, and choose a designated eating area free from clutter. By creating a dedicated space and time for eating, we signal to ourselves that this moment is worthy of our full attention.

Savoring each bite is an integral aspect of mindful eating. It's about fully experiencing the flavors, textures, and sensations of the food. This practice engages all our senses—sight, smell, touch, taste, and even sound. By savoring each bite, we transform eating into a sensory delight. We notice the colors and arrangement of our food, inhale its aroma, and appreciate its presentation. This multisensory experience enhances our connection with the food and elevates the act of eating from mere sustenance to a pleasurable and mindful engagement with our senses.

Mindful drinking extends the principles of mindful eating to beverages. Whether it's water, tea, or coffee, we can apply mindfulness to our drinks. Instead of guzzling down a beverage mindlessly, we take the time to appreciate each sip. We notice the temperature, taste, and sensations as we drink. This practice reinforces the concept that mindfulness can be applied to all aspects of our daily consumption, not just solid foods. Mindful snacking is an extension of the practice beyond formal meals. Rather than mindlessly reaching for a snack in response to boredom or stress, we pause to assess our level of hunger. If we are genuinely hungry, we choose a nutritious snack and savor it with the same mindfulness we apply to meals. This practice helps us differentiate between emotional cravings and genuine hunger, promoting healthier snacking habits. Mindful gratitude is a technique that invites us to pause and express gratitude for the food in front of us. It encourages reflection on the effort that went into its preparation, from farm to table. This practice deepens our connection with our food and instills a sense of appreciation for the sustenance it provides. Gratitude extends beyond the act of eating and can foster a greater awareness of the interconnectedness of food, nature, and the individuals involved in its production. Reflecting on our eating experience is an essential technique for mindful eating. After each meal, we take a moment to contemplate our experience. How did mindful eating make us feel physically and emotionally? What did we learn about our hunger and fullness cues? These reflections deepen our practice over time and provide valuable insights into our relationship with food and our body. They create a feedback loop that enables us to refine our mindful eating skills continually. Cultivating patience with ourselves is fundamental to the practice of mindful eating. Mindfulness is a skill that develops over time, and it is not about achieving perfection but rather about embracing progress and intention. It is natural to encounter challenges along the way, such as moments of mindlessness or lapses in awareness. Instead of self-criticism, we practice self-compassion, recognizing that these challenges are part of the journey. Mindful eating is not a destination but an ongoing process, and the intention to cultivate a more mindful relationship with food is a significant step forward. Mindful eating is a practice that transcends the act of eating; it is a profound shift in the way we relate to food and our bodies. The techniques discussed here empower us to approach meals with intention, presence, and gratitude. They encourage us to slow down, listen to our body's cues, and create an environment conducive to mindfulness. Mindful eating is not a set of rigid rules but a journey of self-discovery and self-compassion. It is an invitation to savor the richness of the present moment, one bite at a time, and to cultivate a profound connection with the nourishment that sustains us.

Overcoming Emotional Eating

Emotional eating is a complex and often challenging pattern of behavior that many individuals grapple with. It occurs when people turn to food as a way to cope with their emotions, rather than eating for physical hunger or nourishment. These emotions can range from stress and anxiety to sadness, boredom, or even joy. Emotional eating can become a habitual response to life's ups and downs, leading to a cycle of overeating, guilt, and dissatisfaction. However, it is possible to overcome emotional eating and develop healthier ways of coping with emotions. One essential step in overcoming emotional eating is self-awareness. It begins with recognizing and acknowledging the triggers that lead to emotional eating episodes. These triggers can vary widely from person to person and may include stress at work, relationship issues, financial worries, or even positive events like celebrations. By identifying these triggers, individuals can start to understand the emotional patterns that drive their eating behavior. Journaling or keeping a food diary can be helpful in tracking emotional eating episodes and identifying the underlying emotions and situations that precede them. Once the triggers are identified, it's crucial to develop alternative coping mechanisms for dealing with these emotions. This involves building a toolbox of healthy strategies to replace emotional eating. These strategies can include exercise, meditation, deep breathing exercises, mindfulness techniques, or engaging in hobbies and activities that bring joy and relaxation. The goal is to redirect the impulse to eat when stressed or upset towards more constructive ways of managing emotions. Developing these coping mechanisms may take time and practice, but they are invaluable in breaking the cycle of emotional eating. Building emotional resilience is another critical aspect of overcoming emotional eating. This involves developing the ability to manage and cope with challenging emotions in a healthier manner. Cognitive-behavioral therapy (CBT) can be particularly effective in helping individuals recognize and change thought patterns that contribute to emotional eating. By challenging and reframing negative thoughts and beliefs about food and emotions, CBT helps individuals develop healthier responses to emotional triggers. Mindful eating practices are invaluable tools in overcoming emotional eating. Mindfulness encourages individuals to become fully present in the eating experience, focusing on the sensory aspects of food, such as taste, texture, and smell. By practicing mindfulness, individuals can develop a greater awareness of physical hunger and fullness cues, making it easier to distinguish between true hunger and emotional eating. Mindful eating also helps individuals savor their food and cultivate a more positive relationship with what they eat. Addressing emotional eating often involves examining and challenging the role of food in one's life. For some, food may have become a primary source of comfort, reward, or stress relief. It's essential to explore these emotional connections to food and work on changing them. This may include reframing the way food is perceived, viewing it primarily as nourishment rather than a means of emotional escape. Nutrition education can also be beneficial in helping individuals make healthier food choices and understand the nutritional impact of their eating habits. Social support is a vital component of overcoming emotional eating. Sharing one's struggles with trusted friends, family members, or support groups can provide emotional validation and encouragement. It can also be helpful to seek the guidance of a therapist or counselor who specializes in emotional eating and can provide tailored strategies and support. The journey to overcoming emotional eating can be challenging, but knowing that one is not alone and has a support system can make a significant difference. Stress management techniques play a crucial role in overcoming emotional eating. Stress is a common trigger for emotional eating, and finding effective ways to manage stress is essential. Exercise is a powerful stress reducer and can also help regulate mood by releasing endorphins. Techniques like yoga and meditation can promote relaxation and improve emotional well-being. Additionally, establishing a regular sleep routine and prioritizing sleep is important, as sleep deprivation can exacerbate emotional eating tendencies. Creating a supportive environment for healthy eating is another essential strategy. This involves making changes in one's living space to facilitate better eating habits. It may mean removing tempting, unhealthy foods from the home or replacing them with nutritious alternatives. Stocking the kitchen with whole foods, fruits, vegetables, and lean proteins can make it easier to make healthy choices when the urge to emotionally eat arises. Practicing self-compassion is a key component of overcoming emotional eating. It's crucial to recognize that setbacks are a natural part of the process, and individuals should not be too hard on themselves if they have occasional lapses in their efforts. Instead of self-criticism, individuals can practice self-compassion by acknowledging their efforts to change and treating themselves with kindness and understanding. Negative self-talk and guilt can exacerbate emotional eating, so cultivating self-compassion is an important countermeasure. Seeking professional help may be necessary for individuals struggling with severe emotional eating patterns that are difficult to overcome on their own. Therapists, counselors, and registered dietitians who specialize in emotional eating can provide specialized guidance and support tailored to an individual's unique needs. They may use various therapeutic modalities, including CBT, mindfulness-based approaches, and nutrition education, to address the underlying emotional and psychological factors contributing to emotional eating. Overcoming emotional eating is a journey that requires self-awareness, self-compassion, and the development of healthier coping mechanisms. It's about recognizing the triggers that lead to emotional eating and finding alternative ways to manage emotions. It involves building emotional resilience, practicing mindful eating, and seeking social support. Developing healthier beliefs and attitudes about food, managing stress effectively, and creating a supportive environment for healthy eating are all crucial components of this process. While overcoming emotional eating can be challenging, with determination and the right strategies, individuals can break free from the cycle of emotional eating and cultivate a more positive and balanced relationship with food and emotions.

Chapter 3
Building a Healthy Plate

Portion Control

Portion control is a fundamental aspect of maintaining a healthy and balanced diet. It involves being mindful of the quantity of food we consume during a meal or snack, and it plays a crucial role in managing calorie intake, supporting weight management, and promoting overall well-being. While portion control may seem straightforward, it can be challenging in a society where super-sized meals and oversized servings have become the norm. However, understanding the importance of portion control and learning practical strategies to implement it can have significant benefits for our health. At its core, portion control is about eating the right amount of food to meet our nutritional needs without overindulging. It is not about deprivation or restricting food intake to the point of discomfort but about finding a balance that ensures we receive adequate nutrients while preventing excess calorie consumption. One of the key benefits of portion control is its role in weight management. When we consistently consume larger portions than our bodies require, it can lead to weight gain over time. By moderating portion sizes, we create a calorie deficit that supports weight loss or helps maintain a healthy weight.

Moreover, portion control is instrumental in preventing overeating, which can lead to discomfort, indigestion, and other gastrointestinal issues. Overeating can also disrupt hunger and fullness cues, making it more challenging to recognize genuine hunger and satiety. Portion control helps us tune in to these cues, making it easier to eat when hungry and stop when satisfied. This intuitive approach to eating aligns our dietary choices with our body's natural rhythms and fosters a healthier relationship with food. Practicing portion control is particularly relevant in a culture where larger portions have become the norm. Many restaurants serve oversized meals that far exceed recommended portion sizes, and packaged foods often contain multiple servings per container. This distortion of portion sizes can lead to unintentional overconsumption and contribute to the obesity epidemic. By becoming more mindful of portion sizes and learning to estimate appropriate servings, individuals can make informed choices when dining out or purchasing packaged foods. A fundamental aspect of portion control is understanding what constitutes a standard serving size. Many people are surprised to learn that their perception of a serving size often differs from the recommended guidelines. For example, a single serving of pasta is typically one cup cooked, but many restaurant portions contain several cups. Familiarizing oneself with standard serving sizes for different food groups, such as grains, proteins, fruits, and vegetables, is a valuable starting point for practicing portion control. Practical strategies for implementing portion control can be integrated into daily eating habits. One effective approach is to use smaller plates and utensils. Research has shown that people tend to eat less when they are served on smaller plates, as it creates the illusion of a fuller plate. Additionally, using smaller utensils, such as salad forks instead of dinner forks, can slow down the eating process, allowing more time for satiety signals to register.

Another technique is to measure or weigh portions, at least initially, to gain a better understanding of what an appropriate serving looks like. This can be particularly helpful for foods that are easy to overeat, such as cereal, nuts, or snacks. After a period of measuring, individuals often become better at estimating portion sizes by sight.

Practicing mindful eating is closely related to portion control. It encourages individuals to pay full attention to their eating experience, including the taste, texture, and smell of food. By being present in the moment, individuals can savor each bite and recognize when they are satisfied. Mindful eating also discourages distractions during meals, such as watching television or working, which can lead to mindless overeating.

Understanding calorie density is another valuable aspect of portion control. Calorie density refers to the number of calories in a given volume of food. Foods with lower calorie density, such as fruits, vegetables, and broth-based soups, provide fewer calories for a larger volume. On the other hand, foods with higher calorie density, such as fried foods, sugary snacks, and fatty cuts of meat, pack more calories into a smaller volume. By choosing foods with lower calorie density, individuals can enjoy larger portions while still managing calorie intake effectively.

Practicing portion control also involves being mindful of portion distortions when dining out. Many restaurants serve portions that exceed recommended serving sizes, which can contribute to overeating. To address this, individuals can consider sharing a dish with a dining partner or requesting a half portion when possible. Alternatively, they can ask for a to-go box at the beginning of the meal and set aside a portion to take home before starting to eat.

Label reading is an essential skill for practicing portion control, especially when it comes to packaged foods. Nutrition labels provide information on serving sizes and the number of servings per container. By paying attention to these details, individuals can make informed choices about portion sizes and calorie intake. It's important to note that the serving size listed on the label may differ from what a person typically consumes, so comparing the label's information to one's own serving size is crucial. Incorporating portion control into daily life can have numerous health benefits. It supports weight management by reducing calorie intake, helps prevent overeating and discomfort, and fosters a healthier relationship with food. Additionally, it can be a valuable tool for managing chronic conditions such as diabetes, where portion sizes and carbohydrate intake play a crucial role in blood sugar control. For individuals looking to lose weight, portion control is often an integral component of their dietary plan, helping them create a sustainable calorie deficit.

Portion control is a versatile concept that can be applied to a wide range of dietary preferences and lifestyles. Whether an individual follows a vegetarian, vegan, paleo, or Mediterranean diet, portion control remains relevant. It allows individuals to adapt their dietary choices to align with their specific goals and needs while still enjoying a variety of foods in appropriate amounts. Portion control is a fundamental aspect of a healthy and balanced diet. It involves being mindful of the quantity of food consumed and plays a crucial role in managing calorie intake, supporting weight management, and promoting overall well-being. Practicing portion control includes using smaller plates and utensils, measuring or weighing portions when necessary, practicing mindful eating, understanding calorie density, and being aware of portion distortions when dining out. By incorporating these strategies into daily eating habits, individuals can make informed choices about portion sizes, cultivate a healthier relationship with food, and enjoy the benefits of portion control for their physical and emotional well-being.

Balancing Your Meals

Balancing your meals is a foundational aspect of maintaining a healthy and nutritious diet. It involves the careful consideration and combination of various food groups and nutrients to provide the body with the essential components it needs to function optimally. A balanced meal not only supports overall health but also helps regulate energy levels, stabilize blood sugar, and promote satiety, ultimately contributing to a sense of well-being.

One fundamental principle of balanced meals is the inclusion of macronutrients, namely carbohydrates, proteins, and fats, in appropriate proportions. Carbohydrates are a primary source of energy, providing glucose that fuels the body and brain. Whole grains, fruits, vegetables, and legumes are excellent sources of complex carbohydrates that offer sustained energy. Proteins are essential for tissue repair, immune function, and the production of enzymes and hormones. Including lean proteins such as poultry, fish, tofu, legumes, and dairy products can help meet these nutritional needs. Fats are necessary for the absorption of fat-soluble vitamins and provide a concentrated source of energy. Healthy fats from sources like avocados, nuts, seeds, and olive oil should be part of a balanced meal. In addition to macronutrients, fiber plays a critical role in meal balance. Fiber is primarily found in plant-based foods and offers various health benefits, including improved digestion and enhanced satiety. Fiber-rich foods such as whole grains, fruits, vegetables, and legumes not only provide essential nutrients but also promote digestive health and help regulate blood sugar levels. Incorporating these foods into meals can contribute to a sense of fullness and satisfaction, reducing the likelihood of overeating. Balancing meals also involves paying attention to portion sizes. The appropriate portion size varies depending on individual factors such as age, activity level, and specific dietary goals. However, a general guideline is to fill half of your plate with vegetables and fruits, one-quarter with lean protein sources, and one-quarter with whole grains or starchy vegetables. This visual representation can help individuals gauge whether their meals are proportionally balanced and aligned with their nutritional needs. Variety is a cornerstone of balanced meals. Including a wide range of foods not only ensures a diverse intake of nutrients but also makes meals more enjoyable. Different food groups offer distinct vitamins, minerals, and phytonutrients, and consuming a variety of foods can help prevent nutritional deficiencies and promote overall health. An emphasis on colorful fruits and vegetables, in particular, ensures a broad spectrum of antioxidants and other beneficial compounds that support well-being. Balanced meals also account for individual dietary preferences and restrictions. Whether someone follows a vegetarian, vegan, gluten-free, or other dietary pattern, it's essential to adapt meal planning to meet their specific nutritional needs. For instance, plant-based diets can provide ample nutrients when carefully balanced, ensuring sufficient protein, vitamins, and minerals. Similarly, gluten-free diets can be balanced by incorporating naturally gluten-free whole grains like rice, quinoa, and oats. Mindful eating practices are closely related to balanced meals. Eating mindfully involves being fully present during meals, savoring each bite, and paying attention to hunger and fullness cues. By practicing mindfulness, individuals can become attuned to their body's signals and make more conscious choices about portion sizes and food selection. This approach encourages a deeper appreciation for the sensory experience of eating and fosters a positive relationship with food. Timing is another aspect of balanced meals that should not be overlooked. Spacing meals and snacks throughout the day can help regulate energy levels and prevent excessive hunger that may lead to overeating. It's essential to listen to the body's natural hunger cues and not skip meals, as this can disrupt metabolism and lead to erratic eating patterns. Additionally, incorporating healthy snacks between meals can provide sustained energy and prevent extreme hunger that may result in poor food choices. Balancing meals also extends to the consideration of hydration. Adequate water intake is essential for overall health and well-being. Drinking water throughout the day helps maintain proper bodily functions, supports digestion, and can prevent confusion of thirst with hunger. Including beverages like water, herbal teas, and diluted fruit juices as part of a meal can contribute to proper hydration. Furthermore, balanced meals consider the specific nutritional needs of different life stages. For example, children and teenagers have increased energy and nutrient requirements to support growth and development. Meals for this age group should include a variety of nutrient-dense foods, along with age-appropriate portion sizes. On the other hand, older adults may require fewer calories but still need adequate protein, fiber, vitamins, and minerals to support aging and overall health. Balanced meals can also be adapted to address specific health conditions or dietary restrictions. For individuals with diabetes, managing carbohydrate intake and monitoring blood sugar levels is crucial. Meals for diabetics should focus on complex carbohydrates, fiber-rich foods, lean proteins, and healthy fats. Similarly, individuals with food allergies or intolerances should carefully select foods that align with their dietary needs and consider alternatives or substitutions to ensure a balanced meal.

Cultural and culinary preferences also play a significant role in the composition of balanced meals. Traditional dishes from various cultures offer a rich tapestry of flavors and ingredients, often incorporating locally available foods and culinary techniques. Embracing these cultural preferences can make meal planning more enjoyable and promote the consumption of a diverse range of foods. Balanced meals promote not only physical but also emotional and psychological well-being. They contribute to a sense of satisfaction and contentment after eating, reducing the likelihood of cravings or overindulgence. By providing essential nutrients and maintaining stable blood sugar levels, balanced meals can help stabilize mood and energy throughout the day. This, in turn, supports cognitive function and overall mental well-being.

Balanced meals are a cornerstone of a healthy diet and overall well-being. They involve the thoughtful combination of macronutrients, fiber, portion sizes, and a wide variety of foods to ensure the body receives the nutrients it needs to function optimally. Balancing meals is not only about physical health but also about embracing cultural preferences, addressing dietary restrictions, and practicing mindful eating. By incorporating these principles into daily meal planning, individuals can promote better nutrition, maintain stable energy levels, and support their long-term health and wellness goals.

The Plate Method

The Plate Method is a practical and visual approach to meal planning that promotes balanced and healthy eating. It's a versatile tool that can help individuals make informed choices about portion sizes and food group distribution, ultimately supporting overall well-being. This method is particularly helpful for those looking to manage their weight, control blood sugar levels, or simply adopt a more balanced diet. The core concept of the Plate Method is to envision your plate as a guide for composing balanced meals. Instead of relying on complex measurements or calorie counting, you use your plate as a visual aid to ensure that you're getting a mix of nutrients and portion sizes that align with your dietary goals. It's a straightforward and flexible approach that can be tailored to various dietary preferences and needs. The Plate Method typically divides the plate into three sections: one-half for vegetables and fruits, one-quarter for lean proteins, and one-quarter for grains or starchy foods. This division not only provides a balanced mix of nutrients but also helps control calorie intake, support healthy blood sugar levels, and encourage portion control. The vegetable and fruit section is a cornerstone of the Plate Method. These foods are rich in essential vitamins, minerals, fiber, and antioxidants, making them essential for overall health. By filling half your plate with vegetables and fruits, you not only increase your intake of these vital nutrients but also naturally limit calorie-dense foods that can contribute to overeating and weight gain. Vegetables and fruits can be fresh, frozen, canned, or dried, allowing for a wide variety of options to suit individual preferences and availability. The lean protein section provides essential amino acids needed for tissue repair, immune function, and overall health. Lean protein sources include poultry, fish, lean cuts of beef or pork, tofu, tempeh, legumes, and dairy products. By dedicating a quarter of your plate to lean proteins, you ensure an adequate intake of these vital nutrients while keeping portion sizes in check. This is particularly important for individuals seeking to manage their weight, as protein can enhance satiety and promote muscle maintenance. The remaining quarter of the plate is allocated to grains or starchy foods. This section provides a source of carbohydrates, which are the body's primary energy source. Whole grains like brown rice, quinoa, whole wheat pasta, and oats are excellent choices as they offer complex carbohydrates, fiber, vitamins, and minerals. Grains and starchy foods are a valuable component of a balanced meal, providing sustained energy and supporting overall dietary satisfaction. In addition to the three main sections, the Plate Method encourages incorporating a source of healthy fat, such as olive oil, nuts, seeds, or avocados. These fats provide essential fatty acids, support the absorption of fat-soluble vitamins, and contribute to satiety. While they aren't assigned a specific portion of the plate, they can be included in the meal as a salad dressing, cooking oil, or a small side portion. The Plate Method is also versatile and adaptable to various dietary preferences and needs. For individuals following vegetarian or vegan diets, the protein section can be filled with plant-based protein sources like tofu, tempeh, legumes, or meat substitutes. Similarly, those with gluten-free diets can select gluten-free grains or starches for the grain section. It's a flexible approach that encourages individuals to choose foods that align with their dietary goals and preferences. Furthermore, the Plate Method can be tailored to specific health conditions or goals. For individuals with diabetes, it can be used as a valuable tool for managing blood sugar levels. By focusing on portion sizes and the distribution of carbohydrates throughout the plate, individuals can create meals that support better glycemic control. Similarly, those looking to manage their weight can use the Plate Method to control calorie intake and support portion control. The visual aspect of the plate makes it easy to gauge portion sizes without the need for detailed measurements. The Plate Method also emphasizes the importance of mindful eating. It encourages individuals to savor each bite, be present in the moment, and pay attention to hunger and fullness cues. By practicing mindful eating, individuals can foster a deeper connection with their food and enhance the overall dining experience. This approach discourages distractions during meals, such as watching television or working, which can lead to mindless overeating.

Incorporating the Plate Method into daily meal planning is relatively straightforward. To get started, individuals can:
1. Choose a suitable plate: Begin with selecting a plate that suits your dietary goals and portion needs. A smaller plate may help

with portion control, while a larger plate can accommodate larger portion sizes if needed.

2. Visualize the plate: Mentally divide the plate into three sections as described earlier: one-half for vegetables and fruits, one-quarter for lean proteins, and one-quarter for grains or starchy foods.

3. Select foods: Fill each section of the plate with foods that correspond to the categories. Choose a variety of vegetables and fruits, opt for lean protein sources, and select whole grains or starchy foods.

4. Add healthy fats: Incorporate a source of healthy fat into the meal, such as olive oil for dressing, nuts as a topping, or avocado as a side dish.

5. Practice portion control: Pay attention to portion sizes within each section of the plate. This may involve measuring or using visual cues to gauge appropriate serving sizes.

6. Enjoy the meal mindfully: Eat slowly and savor each bite. Be present in the moment and pay attention to hunger and fullness cues to determine when you are satisfied.

7. Adapt to dietary preferences: Tailor the Plate Method to suit your dietary preferences, whether you follow a vegetarian, vegan, gluten-free, or other dietary pattern.

The Plate Method is a practical and adaptable approach to meal planning that promotes balanced and healthy eating. By visually dividing the plate into sections for vegetables and fruits, lean proteins, and grains or starchy foods, individuals can create meals that support overall well-being, control calorie intake, and encourage portion control. This method is versatile and can be tailored to various dietary preferences, needs, and health goals. It also promotes mindful eating, fostering a deeper connection with food and enhancing the dining experience. Whether you're looking to manage your weight, control blood sugar levels, or simply adopt a more balanced diet, the Plate Method offers a straightforward and effective way to make informed choices about portion sizes and food group distribution.

Chapter 4
Nourishing Your Body

Eating for Energy and Vitality

Eating for energy and vitality is a fundamental aspect of maintaining a healthy and vibrant lifestyle. The food we consume plays a crucial role in fueling our bodies, supporting our physical and mental well-being, and providing the energy necessary for daily activities. A well-balanced and nutrient-rich diet can boost vitality, enhance productivity, and improve overall quality of life.

One of the primary principles of eating for energy and vitality is selecting a wide variety of nutrient-dense foods. Nutrient-dense foods are those that provide a high concentration of essential vitamins, minerals, antioxidants, and other beneficial compounds relative to their calorie content. These foods include fruits, vegetables, whole grains, lean proteins, nuts, seeds, and dairy products. By prioritizing nutrient-dense foods, individuals can ensure that their bodies receive the essential nutrients necessary for optimal health and vitality. The consumption of fruits and vegetables is particularly critical for energy and vitality. These foods are rich in vitamins, such as vitamin C and vitamin A, as well as minerals like potassium and magnesium, which are essential for various physiological processes. Additionally, fruits and vegetables are abundant sources of antioxidants, which help protect cells from oxidative stress and support overall well-being. A diet rich in colorful fruits and vegetables not only enhances vitality but also reduces the risk of chronic diseases. Another essential aspect of eating for energy and vitality is maintaining stable blood sugar levels. Fluctuations in blood sugar can lead to energy crashes and mood swings. To achieve stable blood sugar levels, individuals should focus on consuming complex carbohydrates, such as whole grains, legumes, and vegetables, which provide a steady release of glucose into the bloodstream. Pairing carbohydrates with lean proteins and healthy fats can further stabilize blood sugar and promote lasting energy. Lean proteins are vital for muscle health and overall vitality. Protein is essential for tissue repair, immune function, and the production of enzymes and hormones. Incorporating lean protein sources like poultry, fish, tofu, beans, and low-fat dairy products into meals supports muscle maintenance and provides a sustained source of energy. Adequate protein intake can also enhance satiety, reducing the likelihood of overeating and promoting a balanced diet. Healthy fats are another key component of eating for energy and vitality. Fats are a concentrated source of energy, providing more than twice the calories per gram compared to carbohydrates and protein. However, not all fats are created equal. Healthy fats, such as those found in avocados, nuts, seeds, and olive oil, offer essential fatty acids, support the absorption of fat-soluble vitamins, and contribute to satiety. Including these fats in the diet can help maintain energy levels throughout the day. Hydration is a fundamental aspect of vitality. Even mild dehydration can lead to feelings of fatigue and reduced cognitive function. Staying well-hydrated supports proper bodily functions, including circulation, digestion, and temperature regulation. Water is the most effective way to maintain hydration, but other beverages like herbal teas and diluted fruit juices can also contribute to fluid intake. The Institute of Medicine recommends an average daily water intake of about 3.7 liters for men and 2.7 liters for women, but individual needs may vary. Meal timing is a crucial consideration when eating for energy and vitality. It's important to distribute meals and snacks throughout the day to maintain stable energy levels and prevent excessive hunger. Skipping meals or going for long periods without food can lead to energy crashes and overeating later in the day. Eating regular, balanced meals and incorporating healthy snacks between meals can provide a sustained source of energy and promote overall well-being. Mindful eating practices are closely related to eating for energy and vitality. Mindful eating involves being fully present during meals, savoring each bite, and paying attention to hunger and fullness cues. By practicing mindfulness, individuals can become more attuned to their body's signals and make conscious choices about portion sizes and food selection. This approach encourages a deeper appreciation for the sensory experience of eating and fosters a positive relationship with food. Incorporating whole foods into the diet is a fundamental aspect of eating for energy and vitality. Whole foods are minimally processed and retain their natural nutrients and fiber content. They include foods like whole grains, fresh fruits and vegetables, lean proteins, and unprocessed nuts and seeds. Whole foods are not only more nutrient-dense but also offer a more sustained source of energy compared to highly processed foods, which are often high in added sugars and unhealthy fats. The role of caffeine and stimulants in energy and vitality is a subject of debate. While caffeine can provide a temporary boost in alertness and energy, it is not a sustainable solution for long-term vitality. Excessive caffeine intake can lead to energy crashes, sleep disturbances, and increased heart rate. Instead of relying on caffeine, individuals seeking sustained energy should prioritize a balanced diet, adequate hydration, regular physical activity, and adequate sleep. Incorporating regular physical activity into one's routine is essential for maintaining energy and vitality. Exercise enhances cardiovascular health, boosts circulation, improves oxygen delivery to tissues, and increases energy levels. Engaging in regular physical activity can also help combat feelings of fatigue and enhance overall well-being. It's important to find an activity or exercise routine that aligns with individual preferences and goals, whether it's walking, cycling, yoga, or strength training. Another critical aspect of eating for energy and vitality is getting enough restorative sleep. Sleep plays a fundamental role in energy regulation, mood stability, and cognitive function. Adults should aim for seven to nine hours of quality sleep per night to support overall well-being. Establishing a consistent sleep routine, creating a comfortable sleep environment, and managing stress can all contribute to better sleep quality and enhanced vitality. Managing stress and practicing relaxation techniques are essential components of maintaining energy and vitality. Chronic stress can lead to feelings of fatigue, emotional exhaustion, and reduced overall well-being. Techniques such as meditation, deep breathing exercises, and mindfulness practices can help manage stress levels and promote a sense of calm and vitality. Regular stress management can also enhance sleep quality, improve mood, and support overall health. Lastly, it's important to address individual dietary preferences and dietary restrictions when eating for energy and vitality. Whether someone follows a vegetarian, vegan, gluten-free, or other dietary pattern, it's essential to adapt meal planning to meet their specific nutritional needs. A well-balanced and nutrient-rich diet can be achieved within various dietary preferences, ensuring that individuals can maintain energy and vitality while aligning with their dietary choices. Eating for energy and vitality involves making conscious choices about the foods we consume, the timing of our meals, and our overall lifestyle. A diet rich in nutrient-dense foods, including fruits, vegetables, lean proteins, and healthy fats, supports optimal health and vitality. Stable blood sugar levels, hydration, regular physical activity, and restorative sleep are all essential components of vitality. Mindful eating practices and stress management techniques also play a vital role in maintaining energy and overall well-being. By prioritizing these aspects of a healthy lifestyle, individuals can experience increased vitality, enhanced productivity, and an improved quality of life.

Choosing Nutrient-Dense Foods

Choosing nutrient-dense foods is a foundational principle of maintaining a healthy and balanced diet. Nutrient density refers to the concentration of essential vitamins, minerals, antioxidants, and other beneficial compounds in a food relative to its calorie content. Nutrient-dense foods provide a wide array of essential nutrients while offering relatively few calories. Making informed choices to prioritize these foods can have a profound impact on overall health and well-being. Vegetables and fruits are exemplary examples of nutrient-dense foods. They are rich sources of vitamins, such as vitamin C, vitamin A, and various B vitamins, along with essential minerals like potassium and magnesium. Additionally, vegetables and fruits are abundant in antioxidants, which help protect cells from oxidative damage. By incorporating a variety of colorful vegetables and fruits into the diet, individuals can boost their intake of essential nutrients, support immune function, and reduce the risk of chronic diseases. Whole grains are another important category of nutrient-dense foods. Unlike refined grains, whole grains retain their bran and germ, which contain a wealth of nutrients and fiber. Nutrients like B vitamins, iron, magnesium, and dietary fiber are essential for overall health. Whole grains such as brown rice, quinoa, whole wheat pasta, and oats provide sustained energy and promote digestive health. They also help stabilize blood sugar levels, reducing the risk of energy crashes and mood swings. Lean proteins are vital for muscle health and overall well-being. Nutrient-dense sources of lean protein include poultry, fish, lean cuts of beef or pork, tofu, tempeh, legumes, and low-fat dairy products. Proteins provide essential amino acids needed for tissue repair, immune function, and the production of enzymes and hormones. Incorporating lean proteins into meals not only supports muscle maintenance but also enhances satiety, reducing the likelihood of overeating and promoting a balanced diet. Nuts and seeds are nutrient-dense sources of healthy fats, vitamins, minerals, and antioxidants. They provide essential fatty acids, such as omega-3 and omega-6 fatty acids, which are crucial for overall health. Nuts like almonds, walnuts, and cashews, along with seeds like chia seeds, flaxseeds, and pumpkin seeds, offer a concentrated source of energy and can contribute to satiety. These foods are versatile and can be incorporated into a wide range of dishes or enjoyed as snacks. Dairy products, such as yogurt, milk, and cheese, are nutrient-dense sources of essential nutrients like calcium, vitamin D, and protein. Calcium is vital for bone health, while vitamin D supports calcium absorption and overall immune function. Opting for low-fat or reduced-fat dairy products can provide these essential nutrients without excess saturated fat and calories. Incorporating dairy into the diet can promote strong bones, support muscle function, and enhance overall nutritional intake. Fish and seafood are exceptional sources of lean protein and essential omega-3 fatty acids, particularly eicosapentaenoic acid (EPA) and docosahexaenoic acid (DHA). Omega-3 fatty acids play a critical role in cardiovascular health, brain function, and inflammation control. Fatty fish like salmon, mackerel, and sardines are especially rich in these beneficial fats. Regular consumption of fish and seafood can reduce the risk of heart disease, support cognitive function, and promote overall well-being. Legumes, which include beans, lentils, chickpeas, and peas, are nutrient-dense plant-based protein sources. They are rich in essential nutrients like folate, iron, potassium, and dietary fiber. Legumes provide sustained energy and support digestive health. Additionally, they are low in fat and can be incorporated into a variety of dishes, making them a versatile choice for those seeking plant-based protein options. Regular consumption of legumes can contribute to overall nutritional intake and promote satiety. Eggs are nutrient-dense sources of high-quality protein, essential vitamins, and minerals. They provide important nutrients such as vitamin B12, choline, and selenium. Eggs are particularly rich in essential amino acids, making them a valuable addition to a balanced diet. They can be prepared in numerous ways and offer a versatile and affordable source of essential nutrients. Focusing on nutrient-dense foods also involves reducing the intake of highly processed and calorie-dense foods that offer little nutritional value. Highly processed foods are often high in added sugars, unhealthy fats, and sodium, contributing to excess calorie intake and the risk of chronic diseases. By minimizing the consumption of these foods, individuals can make room for nutrient-dense choices that provide essential nutrients without excess calories. Beverage choices are an important consideration when selecting nutrient-dense foods. Water is the most effective way to maintain hydration and should be the primary beverage of choice. Herbal teas, which are caffeine-free and naturally calorie-free, can also contribute to hydration. Diluted fruit juices and low-fat or fat-free milk can provide essential nutrients without excessive calories when consumed in moderation. However, it's important to limit the consumption of sugary beverages like sodas, energy drinks, and sugary fruit drinks, which provide added sugars and excess calories with minimal nutritional benefit.

Understanding food labels is a valuable skill when choosing nutrient-dense foods. Nutrition labels provide information on serving sizes, calorie content, and the amount of essential nutrients per serving. By carefully reading labels, individuals can make informed choices about the nutritional quality of foods and select those that align with their dietary goals. Paying attention to portion sizes is particularly important, as it ensures that individuals are aware of the calories and nutrients they are consuming. Meal planning and preparation play a significant role in choosing nutrient-dense foods. Planning meals in advance allows individuals to select a variety of nutrient-dense foods and ensure that their dietary choices align with their nutritional needs. Meal preparation also empowers individuals to control portion sizes, reduce the consumption of unhealthy fats, and limit added sugars and sodium. Cooking at home using fresh, whole ingredients provides greater control over the quality and nutritional value of meals.

Choosing nutrient-dense foods is a fundamental aspect of maintaining a healthy and balanced diet. Nutrient-dense foods provide essential vitamins, minerals, antioxidants, and other beneficial compounds while offering relatively few calories. Prioritizing these foods, such as vegetables, fruits, whole grains, lean proteins, nuts, seeds, dairy products, fish, legumes, eggs, and minimizing highly processed and calorie-dense foods, can have a significant impact on overall health and well-being. Making informed choices, reading food labels, and planning and preparing meals can empower individuals to select nutrient-dense foods that support their dietary goals and promote optimal health.

The Benefits of Hydration

Hydration is a fundamental aspect of maintaining overall health and well-being, and its benefits extend far beyond quenching your thirst. Water is essential for the proper functioning of virtually every system in the human body. It plays a crucial role in digestion, circulation, temperature regulation, and waste elimination. In this comprehensive exploration of the benefits of hydration, we'll delve into the various ways staying adequately hydrated positively impacts your body and overall quality of life. Starting with a fundamental aspect, hydration supports proper bodily functions. Water is the primary component of cells, tissues, and organs. It serves as a medium for chemical reactions, facilitating the transport of nutrients and oxygen to cells while helping remove waste products and toxins from the body. This fundamental role ensures that your body operates efficiently, allowing you to feel your best both physically and mentally. When it comes to maintaining a healthy body weight, hydration plays a significant role. Proper hydration can help control appetite and portion sizes, as thirst can sometimes be mistaken for hunger. Drinking water before or with meals can help you feel more satisfied, reducing the likelihood of overeating and supporting weight management. Additionally, adequate hydration supports metabolic processes, contributing to optimal calorie burning and energy expenditure. Maintaining good cardiovascular health is another critical benefit of hydration. Dehydration can lead to a drop in blood volume, causing the heart to work harder to pump blood and deliver oxygen to the body's cells. Over time, chronic dehydration can contribute to increased strain on the heart and potentially lead to cardiovascular issues. Staying well-hydrated helps maintain blood volume, allowing the heart to function more efficiently and reducing the risk of heart-related problems. Hydration also plays a role in temperature regulation and physical performance. When you exercise or engage in physical activities, your body generates heat. Sweating is the body's natural cooling mechanism, but it also leads to fluid loss. Dehydration can impair your ability to regulate body temperature, making you more susceptible to overheating during exercise. Proper hydration helps maintain thermal regulation, enabling you to perform better and reduce the risk of heat-related illnesses. Cognitive function and mental well-being are closely tied to hydration. Even mild dehydration can negatively impact mood, concentration, and cognitive performance. Research has shown that dehydration can impair memory, attention, and decision-making skills. Staying well-hydrated supports mental clarity, alertness, and overall cognitive function, enhancing your ability to think clearly and maintain focus throughout the day. The importance of hydration in digestion cannot be overstated. Water is a key component in the digestive process, helping break down food, absorb nutrients, and move waste through the digestive tract. Insufficient hydration can lead to constipation, indigestion, and other digestive issues. By drinking enough water, you ensure that your digestive system functions smoothly, promoting regular bowel movements and optimal nutrient absorption. One of the most recognized benefits of hydration is the positive impact it has on the skin's appearance and health. Dehydrated skin can become dry, flaky, and prone to irritation and wrinkles. Drinking enough water helps maintain skin's elasticity and moisture balance, contributing to a more youthful and radiant complexion. While water alone won't solve all skin issues, it plays a crucial role in overall skin health. Hydration is also essential for kidney function. The kidneys play a pivotal role in filtering waste products and excess substances from the blood to form urine. Proper hydration ensures that the kidneys can effectively perform this function, preventing the buildup of toxins and waste in the body. Dehydration can lead to kidney stones and urinary tract infections, which can be painful and disruptive to overall health. Maintaining joint health is yet another benefit of hydration. The synovial fluid that surrounds and lubricates joints is primarily composed of water. Staying adequately hydrated helps ensure that joints function smoothly, reducing the risk of stiffness, discomfort, and injury. Proper hydration is particularly important for individuals with conditions like osteoarthritis, where joint health is already compromised.

For those who engage in regular physical activity or sports, staying hydrated is crucial to performance and recovery. Dehydration can lead to muscle cramps, fatigue, and decreased endurance. Proper hydration helps maintain muscle function, prevent cramps, and reduce the risk of injuries. After exercise, adequate hydration aids in the recovery process, facilitating the repair of muscle tissues and reducing post-workout soreness. Hydration also supports the immune system. The body's immune response relies on the circulation of immune cells and antibodies throughout the body. Dehydration can lead to reduced blood volume and circulation, potentially impairing the immune system's ability to function effectively. Staying well-hydrated helps ensure optimal immune function, supporting the body's ability to defend against illnesses and infections. Good oral health is closely tied to hydration. Saliva plays a critical role in preventing tooth decay and maintaining gum health. When you're adequately hydrated, your body can produce enough saliva to rinse away food particles, neutralize acids, and protect the teeth and gums. Dehydration can lead to dry mouth, which can increase the risk of dental issues such as cavities and gum disease. Hydration is particularly important during pregnancy. Pregnant women require more fluids to support the increased blood volume, amniotic fluid, and the needs of the growing fetus. Dehydration during pregnancy can lead to complications such as preterm labor, urinary tract infections, and an increased risk of heat-related issues. Staying well-hydrated is essential to support a healthy pregnancy and fetal development. The elderly are also at greater risk of dehydration due to various factors, including reduced thirst sensation and kidney function. Dehydration in older adults can lead to confusion, falls, urinary tract infections, and other health complications. Encouraging and assisting older adults in maintaining proper hydration is essential for their overall well-being and quality of life. Hydration plays a role in managing certain medical conditions. For individuals with diabetes, proper hydration can help control blood sugar levels and reduce the risk of complications. Similarly, individuals with kidney stones may be advised to increase fluid intake to help flush out minerals and prevent stone formation. Those with urinary tract infections may benefit from increased hydration to promote the elimination of bacteria. In summary, the benefits of hydration extend far beyond quenching your thirst. Adequate hydration is essential for the proper functioning of every system in the body. It supports digestion, circulation, temperature regulation, waste elimination, and overall physical and mental well-being. Staying well-hydrated helps control appetite, maintain cardiovascular health, regulate body temperature, enhance cognitive function, and support joint health. Proper hydration also promotes healthy skin, kidney function, oral health, and immune function. Whether you're an athlete, pregnant, elderly, or managing a medical condition, staying adequately hydrated is a crucial aspect of maintaining optimal health and quality of life.

Chapter 5
Food and Your Mood

The Gut-Brain Connection

The gut-brain connection, often referred to as the gut-brain axis, is a complex and intricate communication network that links the gastrointestinal system with the central nervous system. This connection plays a fundamental role in regulating various aspects of our health, including digestion, mood, cognitive function, and even immune responses. In recent years, research into this connection has unveiled the profound impact it has on our overall well-being. At the core of the gut-brain connection is the vagus nerve, a long and winding nerve that runs from the brainstem down into the abdomen. This nerve serves as a two-way highway, transmitting signals between the brain and the gut. It allows the brain to send instructions to the digestive system, regulating processes such as stomach acid secretion, digestion, and nutrient absorption. Conversely, it also enables the gut to send signals to the brain, conveying information about its state, including the presence of food, potential threats (such as pathogens), and overall gut health. The gut is home to a vast community of microorganisms collectively referred to as the gut microbiota or gut microbiome. These microbes include bacteria, viruses, fungi, and other microorganisms. The composition and diversity of the gut microbiota play a pivotal role in the gut-brain connection. These microorganisms interact with the gut lining, influencing the production of neurotransmitters, hormones, and other signaling molecules that can affect mood and cognitive function. One of the key ways in which the gut microbiota influences the brain is through the production of neurotransmitters. For example, certain gut bacteria are involved in the synthesis of serotonin, a neurotransmitter that plays a crucial role in regulating mood and is often referred to as the "feel-good" neurotransmitter. Imbalances in the gut microbiota have been linked to alterations in serotonin levels, which can contribute to mood disorders such as depression and anxiety. Moreover, the gut-brain connection plays a significant role in immune system regulation. The gut is the body's largest immune organ, and its microbiota helps train and modulate the immune response. A healthy gut microbiome contributes to a balanced and well-regulated immune system, while disruptions in the gut can lead to inflammation and immune-related conditions. This immune-gut-brain interaction is particularly relevant in the context of autoimmune diseases and conditions like irritable bowel syndrome (IBS) where both gut and mood symptoms are common. The gut-brain connection also influences stress responses and the body's ability to manage stress. The gut communicates with the brain through various signaling molecules, including hormones and peptides. The presence of stressors, whether physical or psychological, can trigger changes in the gut, affecting motility, blood flow, and the balance of the gut microbiota. This can lead to gastrointestinal symptoms in response to stress, a phenomenon often referred to as "nervous stomach" or "butterflies in the stomach."

The gut-brain connection has profound implications for mental health. Numerous studies have shown that the gut microbiota can influence mood and behavior. For example, research in the emerging field of psychobiotics explores the use of specific probiotics or prebiotics to support mental health by modulating the gut microbiome. These interventions hold promise for conditions such as depression, anxiety, and stress-related disorders. The gut-brain connection is also intimately involved in regulating appetite and body weight. Hormones produced in the gut, such as ghrelin and leptin, signal hunger and fullness to the brain. Alterations in gut microbiota composition can impact the regulation of these hormones, potentially contributing to overeating and weight gain. This connection underscores the importance of a balanced gut microbiome in maintaining healthy eating patterns and body weight. Furthermore, recent research suggests that the gut-brain connection may play a role in neurodegenerative diseases such as Alzheimer's and Parkinson's disease. The gut microbiota and the substances they produce can influence neuroinflammation and the aggregation of abnormal proteins in the brain, which are hallmark features of these diseases. While this area of research is still evolving, it highlights the potential for therapeutic interventions targeting the gut to mitigate the progression of neurodegenerative disorders. The gut-brain connection is not a one-size-fits-all phenomenon. It is influenced by various factors, including genetics, diet, lifestyle, and early life experiences. The gut microbiota composition can vary significantly from person to person, and even small changes in diet or environment can have a profound impact on the gut-brain axis. Diet, in particular, plays a critical role in shaping the gut microbiota and, consequently, the gut-brain connection. A diet rich in fiber, whole grains, fruits, and vegetables promotes the growth of beneficial gut bacteria, contributing to a balanced and diverse microbiome. On the other hand, a diet high in processed foods, added sugars, and unhealthy fats can disrupt the gut microbiota and negatively affect the gut-brain axis. Probiotics and prebiotics, which are substances that support the growth of beneficial gut bacteria, have gained attention for their potential to enhance the gut-brain connection. Probiotics are live microorganisms found in fermented foods and supplements, while prebiotics are non-digestible fibers that serve as food for beneficial gut bacteria. These interventions can help restore and maintain a healthy gut microbiome, potentially leading to improvements in mood, cognition, and overall well-being. Stress management techniques also play a crucial role in supporting the gut-brain connection. Chronic stress can disrupt the gut microbiota and exacerbate gastrointestinal symptoms. Practicing stress reduction strategies such as mindfulness, meditation, and deep breathing exercises can help mitigate the negative effects of stress on the gut-brain axis. The gut-brain connection is a fascinating and dynamic communication network that influences various aspects of our health and well-being. It highlights the intricate relationship between the gut, the gut microbiota, and the brain, emphasizing their collective impact on digestion, mood, cognition, immune function, and more. Understanding and nurturing this connection through a balanced diet, stress management, and potentially interventions like probiotics and prebiotics offer exciting possibilities for enhancing mental and physical health. As research continues to unfold, the gut-brain connection promises to be an exciting frontier in the field of health and wellness.

Foods that Boost Mood and Mental Health

The relationship between food and mood is a complex and fascinating one. Research has shown that the foods we eat can have a significant impact on our mental health and emotional well-being. While there is no magic "happy meal," a balanced and nutrient-rich diet can help support mood regulation, reduce the risk of mood disorders, and promote overall mental well-being. At the core of foods that boost mood and mental health is the influence of nutrients on brain function. Nutrients such as vitamins, minerals, amino acids, and fatty acids are essential for the production and regulation of neurotransmitters, which are the brain's chemical messengers. These neurotransmitters play a critical role in mood regulation, cognitive function, and emotional well-being. One of the key nutrients involved in mood regulation is tryptophan, an amino acid found in various protein-rich foods. Tryptophan is a precursor to serotonin, a neurotransmitter often referred to as the "feel-good" neurotransmitter. Consuming foods rich in tryptophan, such as turkey, chicken, fish, eggs, nuts, and seeds, can support serotonin production and contribute to a more positive mood. Another essential nutrient for mood and mental health is omega-3 fatty acids, particularly EPA (eicosapentaenoic acid) and DHA (docosahexaenoic acid). These fatty acids are abundant in fatty fish like salmon, mackerel, and sardines, as well as in flaxseeds, chia seeds, and walnuts. Omega-3s play a crucial role in reducing inflammation in the brain, which has been linked to mood disorders such as depression. Regular consumption of omega-3-rich foods can help support a stable and positive mood. Antioxidants, found in fruits and vegetables, play a vital role in protecting the brain from oxidative stress and inflammation. Oxidative stress can damage brain cells and contribute to mood disorders. Foods rich in antioxidants, such as berries, leafy greens, and colorful vegetables, provide protection against this damage and support overall brain health. B vitamins, including folate, B6, and B12, are essential for neurotransmitter production and regulation. Low levels of these vitamins have been associated with an increased risk of depression and other mood disorders. Foods like leafy greens, legumes, fortified cereals, and lean meats are excellent sources of B vitamins and can support a balanced mood. Amino acids like tyrosine and phenylalanine are precursors to dopamine and norepinephrine, neurotransmitters that play a role in motivation and focus. Foods rich in these amino acids, such as lean meats, dairy products, tofu, and nuts, can contribute to mental alertness and a positive outlook. Magnesium is a mineral that plays a crucial role in nerve function and mood regulation. Inadequate magnesium intake has been linked to an increased risk of depression and anxiety. Foods rich in magnesium, such as leafy greens, nuts, seeds, and whole grains, can support mood stability and overall mental health. The gut-brain connection, as mentioned earlier, also plays a significant role in mood and mental health. A balanced and diverse gut microbiome, influenced by dietary choices, can positively impact the gut-brain axis. Fermented foods like yogurt, kefir, sauerkraut, and kimchi contain beneficial probiotics that promote gut health and, in turn, may support mood and emotional well-being.

It's important to note that while certain foods can support mood and mental health, there is no single "magic" food that can cure or prevent mental health disorders. Rather, it's the overall dietary pattern that matters. A well-balanced diet that includes a variety of nutrient-rich foods provides the essential building blocks for a healthy brain and positive mood. The Mediterranean diet, for example, is often associated with improved mental well-being. This diet emphasizes fruits, vegetables, whole grains, legumes, nuts, seeds, and olive oil, while also including moderate amounts of fish, poultry, and dairy. The combination of nutrient-dense foods, healthy fats, and antioxidants in the Mediterranean diet can support mood regulation and reduce the risk of mood disorders. In contrast, a diet high in processed foods, added sugars, unhealthy fats, and low in nutrients can have a negative impact on mental health. Studies have shown that the consumption of a Western-style diet, characterized by fast food, sugary drinks, and highly processed foods, is associated with an increased risk of depression and anxiety. The timing and frequency of meals can also influence mood and mental health. Skipping meals or going long periods without eating can lead to fluctuations in blood sugar levels, which can contribute to mood swings and irritability. Regular and balanced meals and snacks throughout the day help maintain stable blood sugar levels, providing a consistent source of energy for the brain. Hydration is another crucial aspect of mood and mental health. Dehydration can lead to symptoms such as fatigue, difficulty concentrating, and mood disturbances. Staying adequately hydrated supports cognitive function and emotional well-being. Water is the best choice for hydration, but herbal teas and diluted fruit juices can also contribute to fluid intake.

In addition to specific nutrients and dietary patterns, mindful eating practices can promote a positive relationship with food and support mental well-being. Mindful eating involves being fully present during meals, savoring each bite, and paying attention to hunger and fullness cues. By practicing mindfulness, individuals can develop a healthier and more balanced approach to eating, reducing the risk of emotional eating and promoting a positive body image. The connection between food and mood is undeniable. Nutrient-rich foods provide the essential building blocks for neurotransmitter production, brain function, and mood regulation. A balanced diet that includes a variety of fruits, vegetables, whole grains, lean proteins, healthy fats, and probiotic-rich foods can support mental well-being. On the other hand, a diet high in processed foods, added sugars, and unhealthy fats can have a negative impact on mood and increase the risk of mood disorders. Incorporating mindful eating practices and maintaining adequate hydration further enhance the positive effects of a healthy diet on mental health. While food alone cannot replace professional mental health treatment, it is a valuable tool for promoting emotional well-being and maintaining a positive outlook on life.

Strategies for Reducing Stress Eating

Stress eating, also known as emotional eating, is a common response to stress, anxiety, and other emotional triggers. It involves consuming food, often unhealthy or comfort foods, as a way to cope with emotional distress. While occasional stress eating is normal, it can become problematic when it becomes a habitual response to stress, leading to weight gain, poor nutrition, and emotional reliance on food. Fortunately, there are effective strategies for reducing stress eating and developing healthier coping mechanisms. One of the first steps in addressing stress eating is building awareness. It's essential to recognize when stress eating occurs and identify the emotional triggers that lead to it. Keep a food journal to track eating patterns and note the circumstances and emotions associated with stress eating episodes. This self-awareness can help you identify patterns and gain insight into your emotional relationship with food. Mindfulness techniques are valuable tools for managing stress eating. Mindfulness involves being fully present in the moment, without judgment. When applied to eating, it encourages you to pay close attention to the sensory experience of eating, including taste, texture, and aroma. Practicing mindful eating can help you become more attuned to physical hunger cues and distinguish them from emotional cravings. It can also provide a sense of control over your eating habits, reducing impulsive or emotional eating. Stress management is a crucial component of reducing stress eating. Engaging in stress-reduction activities can help prevent emotional eating in the first place. Regular exercise, such as yoga, meditation, deep breathing exercises, and progressive muscle relaxation, can effectively reduce stress and promote emotional well-being. Finding healthy ways to manage stress, such as these relaxation techniques, can help break the connection between stress and eating. Establishing a structured eating routine can also be beneficial. Regular, balanced meals and snacks at consistent times throughout the day help stabilize blood sugar levels, reducing the likelihood of intense hunger and impulsive eating. Skipping meals or going too long without eating can lead to increased cravings for high-calorie comfort foods. Another strategy for reducing stress eating is to create a supportive environment. Stock your kitchen with nutritious, satisfying snacks and remove or minimize access to highly processed and unhealthy foods. Make it easy to choose healthier options by prepping and portioning fruits, vegetables, and other wholesome snacks in advance. Surrounding yourself with a positive and supportive environment can help reinforce healthier eating habits. Incorporating stress-reducing foods into your diet can also be a helpful strategy. Some foods contain compounds that promote relaxation and reduce stress hormones. For example, foods rich in magnesium, such as nuts, seeds, and leafy greens, can help relax muscles and reduce anxiety. Consuming complex carbohydrates, such as whole grains, can trigger the release of serotonin, a neurotransmitter that promotes a sense of calm. Including stress-reducing foods in your diet can be part of a holistic approach to managing stress eating. Emotional support is essential in addressing stress eating. Connecting with friends, family, or a mental health professional can provide a safe space to discuss your feelings and emotions without turning to food for comfort. Engaging in counseling or therapy can help you develop healthier coping mechanisms for dealing with stress and emotional challenges. Practicing self-care is another vital strategy for reducing stress eating. Self-care activities like taking relaxing baths, reading, spending time in nature, or pursuing hobbies can provide emotional comfort and reduce the need for food as a coping mechanism. Self-care practices promote a sense of well-being and self-compassion, helping to break the cycle of stress eating. Cognitive-behavioral techniques can also be effective in addressing stress eating. Cognitive-behavioral therapy (CBT) focuses on identifying and challenging negative thought patterns and developing healthier behaviors. In the context of stress eating, CBT can help individuals recognize and change the automatic thoughts and beliefs that drive emotional eating. Learning to reframe thoughts and develop healthier coping strategies is a key component of CBT. Creating a support network can provide motivation and accountability in your efforts to reduce stress eating. Sharing your goals and progress with a friend, family member, or support group can offer encouragement and guidance. Additionally, seeking professional support from a registered dietitian or therapist specializing in eating disorders can provide personalized strategies for managing stress eating. Healthy coping mechanisms are essential in replacing stress eating. Identifying alternative ways to deal with stress and emotions can be empowering. Engage in activities that bring joy and relaxation, such as hobbies, art, music, or spending time with loved ones. Physical activity, even a brisk walk, can release endorphins, which are natural mood lifters. Consider keeping a list of activities that bring you happiness and use it as a resource when stress or emotions arise.

Developing a toolkit of stress management techniques is crucial. Experiment with different strategies to determine what works best for you. It may take time and practice to find the most effective methods for managing stress and reducing emotional eating. Remember that stress eating is a learned behavior, and it can be unlearned with patience and persistence. In summary, reducing stress eating involves a multifaceted approach that addresses the emotional, psychological, and behavioral aspects of this habit.

Building awareness of triggers, practicing mindfulness, and engaging in stress management activities are essential steps. Creating a supportive environment, incorporating stress-reducing foods, seeking emotional support, and practicing self-care are additional strategies. Cognitive-behavioral techniques and professional guidance can help reshape thought patterns and behaviors associated with stress eating. Developing healthy coping mechanisms and building a toolbox of stress management techniques ultimately empower individuals to break the cycle of stress eating and nurture a positive relationship with food and emotions.

Chapter 6
Food Allergies and Sensitivities

Understanding Food Allergies

Food allergies are complex and potentially life-threatening immune responses to specific proteins found in certain foods. Unlike food intolerances, which involve difficulty digesting or processing certain substances in food, food allergies are driven by the immune system's reaction to perceived threats. These allergic reactions can range from mild hives or gastrointestinal discomfort to severe anaphylaxis, a rapid and severe reaction that requires immediate medical attention. The immune system plays a pivotal role in protecting the body from harmful invaders, such as bacteria, viruses, and parasites. However, in individuals with food allergies, the immune system mistakenly identifies proteins in certain foods as threats and launches an attack. This immune response triggers the release of various chemicals, including histamines, which lead to allergic symptoms. Common food allergens include peanuts, tree nuts, milk, eggs, soy, wheat, fish, and shellfish. These allergens can be found in a wide range of foods, making it crucial for individuals with food allergies to carefully read labels and inquire about ingredients when dining out. Food allergies can develop at any age, and some children may outgrow their allergies, particularly those to milk, egg, soy, and wheat. The severity of food allergies varies from person to person. Some individuals may experience mild symptoms, such as itching or a runny nose, while others may have severe reactions, including difficulty breathing and a drop in blood pressure. Anaphylaxis, the most severe form of allergic reaction, is a medical emergency that can result in loss of consciousness and death if not treated promptly with epinephrine, a medication that counteracts the effects of the allergic response. Food allergies are diagnosed through a combination of medical history, physical examination, and specific allergy tests. The first step is typically a detailed discussion with a healthcare provider to identify the foods and symptoms involved. Skin prick tests or blood tests, such as the specific IgE test, can help identify food allergies by measuring the presence of allergen-specific antibodies in the blood. In some cases, an oral food challenge, conducted under medical supervision, may be necessary to confirm a diagnosis. One of the most effective ways to manage food allergies is to avoid the allergenic foods. This requires careful label reading, as well as communication with foodservice providers when dining out. Individuals with food allergies often carry epinephrine auto-injectors, such as EpiPen, for emergency use. These devices can be life-saving in the event of an allergic reaction and should be readily accessible at all times. Food allergies can impact not only the individual with the allergy but also their family and social circle. Managing a food allergy requires constant vigilance and communication to ensure that allergenic foods are avoided. Families often need to educate themselves and others about the allergy, as well as develop strategies for safe food preparation and dining. Schools, restaurants, and food manufacturers have also implemented allergen labeling and protocols to protect individuals with food allergies. It's important to distinguish between food allergies and other adverse reactions to food, such as food intolerances and sensitivities. Food intolerances, like lactose intolerance or non-celiac gluten sensitivity, do not involve the immune system and typically result in gastrointestinal symptoms like bloating, diarrhea, or gas. Food sensitivities, on the other hand, may lead to a range of non-specific symptoms, including headaches, fatigue, and joint pain, but are not driven by the immune system. Food allergies are a growing public health concern, with rates on the rise in many parts of the world. The reasons for this increase are not entirely understood but are believed to involve a combination of genetic, environmental, and lifestyle factors. Some theories suggest that early introduction of allergenic foods or alterations in the gut microbiome may contribute to the development of food allergies. However, more research is needed to fully understand these complex mechanisms. There is currently no cure for food allergies, but ongoing research offers hope for potential treatments in the future. One area of study involves desensitization therapies, which aim to gradually expose individuals to small amounts of allergenic foods to reduce their sensitivity. These therapies are still experimental and not widely available, but they hold promise for improving the lives of those with food allergies. In the meantime, the primary management strategy remains strict avoidance of allergenic foods and emergency preparedness in case of accidental exposure. Education and awareness about food allergies are crucial, as is the development of support networks for individuals and families living with these conditions. Food allergies are immune system reactions to specific proteins in certain foods. These allergies can range from mild to severe and can result in life-threatening reactions, known as anaphylaxis. Common allergenic foods include peanuts, tree nuts, milk, eggs, soy, wheat, fish, and shellfish. Diagnosis typically involves medical history, physical examination, and specific allergy tests. Management involves strict avoidance of allergenic foods and emergency preparedness, including carrying epinephrine auto-injectors. The rise in food allergies is a significant public health concern, and ongoing research aims to better understand and treat these conditions. Education, awareness, and support networks are essential for individuals and families living with food allergies.

Identifying Food Sensitivities
Identifying food sensitivities, also known as food intolerances, is a process that involves recognizing adverse reactions to specific foods that do not involve the immune system. Unlike food allergies, which are immune-mediated responses, food sensitivities are characterized by a range of symptoms that can vary widely from person to person. These reactions can affect the gastrointestinal system, skin, or other parts of the body, making it essential to identify and manage them effectively. One common food sensitivity is lactose intolerance, which occurs due to an inability to digest lactose, the sugar found in milk and dairy products, properly. People with lactose intolerance may experience symptoms like bloating, gas, diarrhea, and abdominal discomfort after consuming lactose-containing foods or drinks. This intolerance is caused by a deficiency of lactase, the enzyme required to break down lactose in the digestive system.
Another well-known food sensitivity is non-celiac gluten sensitivity (NCGS). Individuals with NCGS experience symptoms similar to those with celiac disease, such as gastrointestinal discomfort, fatigue, and headaches, when consuming gluten-

containing foods like wheat, barley, and rye. However, unlike celiac disease, NCGS does not involve the immune system and does not result in damage to the small intestine. FODMAP intolerance is a food sensitivity that involves difficulty digesting certain types of carbohydrates known as fermentable oligosaccharides, disaccharides, monosaccharides, and polyols. These carbohydrates are found in a variety of foods, including wheat, certain fruits, vegetables, and dairy products. People with FODMAP intolerance may experience symptoms like abdominal pain, bloating, and diarrhea after consuming high-FODMAP foods. Identifying food sensitivities often begins with self-observation. Individuals may notice that they consistently experience symptoms such as gastrointestinal discomfort, skin issues, headaches, or fatigue after consuming specific foods or food groups. Keeping a food diary can be a valuable tool for tracking symptoms and identifying potential triggers. Elimination diets are a common approach to identifying food sensitivities. This method involves removing suspected trigger foods from the diet for a specified period, typically several weeks. During this elimination phase, individuals carefully monitor their symptoms to see if they improve. After the elimination phase, specific foods are gradually reintroduced, one at a time, while monitoring for the return of symptoms. If symptoms reappear after reintroducing a particular food, it may indicate a sensitivity to that food. In some cases, individuals may seek medical advice to help identify food sensitivities. A healthcare provider can conduct various tests, such as breath tests for lactose or fructose intolerance, blood tests for celiac disease or IgG food intolerance, or skin prick tests for histamine intolerance. However, it's essential to note that some of these tests may have limitations, and their accuracy can vary. A widely recognized method for diagnosing celiac disease is a small intestine biopsy, where a sample of the small intestine is examined for damage caused by gluten consumption. This procedure is typically reserved for individuals suspected of having celiac disease rather than food sensitivities. Once food sensitivities are identified, management strategies can help individuals avoid symptom triggers while maintaining a well-balanced diet. For lactose intolerance, dietary changes may include the consumption of lactose-free dairy products or the use of lactase enzyme supplements before consuming lactose-containing foods. In the case of NCGS, individuals can follow a gluten-free diet, avoiding wheat, barley, and rye products. For those with FODMAP intolerance, a low-FODMAP diet, supervised by a registered dietitian, can help manage symptoms by restricting high-FODMAP foods. It's important to approach food sensitivity identification and management with caution, as self-diagnosis and dietary restrictions can have unintended consequences. Restricting certain foods without professional guidance can lead to nutritional deficiencies, especially when eliminating whole food groups. Therefore, consultation with a healthcare provider or registered dietitian is advisable when attempting to identify and manage food sensitivities. In summary, food sensitivities involve adverse reactions to specific foods or components of foods that do not involve the immune system. Lactose intolerance, non-celiac gluten sensitivity, and FODMAP intolerance are common examples. Identifying food sensitivities typically begins with self-observation and may involve keeping a food diary or trying an elimination diet. Medical tests and consultations with healthcare providers can also aid in diagnosis. Once identified, food sensitivities can be managed through dietary modifications and professional guidance. It's essential to approach the process with care to avoid nutritional deficiencies and ensure a well-balanced diet.

Managing Allergies and Sensitivities in Your Diet

Managing allergies and sensitivities in your diet is a crucial aspect of maintaining your health and well-being. Food allergies and sensitivities can cause a wide range of symptoms, from mild discomfort to severe reactions, and they require careful attention and diligence when it comes to food choices and meal preparation. For individuals with food allergies, the primary focus is on strict avoidance of allergenic foods. This means thoroughly reading food labels to identify potential allergens and communicating dietary restrictions to foodservice providers when dining out. Allergen labeling laws in many countries require manufacturers to clearly indicate the presence of common allergens such as peanuts, tree nuts, milk, eggs, soy, wheat, fish, and shellfish on food labels.

However, it's still essential to check labels carefully, as cross-contamination or hidden sources of allergens can be a concern.

Carrying an epinephrine auto-injector, such as an EpiPen, is often recommended for individuals with severe allergies, as it can be life-saving in the event of an allergic reaction. Epinephrine works quickly to counteract the effects of the allergic response and should be administered immediately if symptoms of anaphylaxis, a severe and potentially life-threatening reaction, occur. In addition to reading labels, individuals with food allergies should be proactive when dining out or attending social events. It's essential to inform restaurant staff or hosts about allergies, ask about ingredients in dishes, and make sure that cross-contamination risks are minimized in food preparation. Many restaurants are trained to accommodate food allergies, but clear communication is key to a safe dining experience. Managing food sensitivities, on the other hand, involves identifying and avoiding specific foods or components that trigger adverse reactions. For example, individuals with lactose intolerance can choose lactose-free dairy products or take lactase enzyme supplements before consuming dairy. Those with non-celiac gluten sensitivity (NCGS) need to avoid wheat, barley, and rye products and opt for gluten-free alternatives. In the case of FODMAP intolerance, individuals may follow a low-FODMAP diet, which restricts fermentable carbohydrates found in various foods. This diet should be done under the guidance of a registered dietitian to ensure nutritional adequacy. Additionally, for those with histamine intolerance, avoiding foods that are high in histamine or trigger histamine release is recommended. When managing food sensitivities, it's essential to maintain a balanced and nutritious diet. Eliminating certain foods or food groups can potentially lead to nutrient deficiencies, so careful planning is necessary. Consulting with a registered dietitian can help individuals create a customized eating plan that meets their nutritional needs while avoiding symptom triggers. It's also important to recognize that the impact of food sensitivities can vary from person to person. Some individuals may have mild reactions to specific foods, while others may experience more severe symptoms. Keeping a food diary can help identify patterns and pinpoint specific trigger foods. In both cases of food allergies and sensitivities, education and awareness are critical.

Individuals with allergies and sensitivities must be well-informed about their condition, understand the symptoms, and know how to respond to allergic reactions or adverse food-related symptoms.

This knowledge empowers them to take control of their diet and make informed choices to safeguard their health. Support networks can be invaluable for those managing allergies and sensitivities. Family members, friends, and coworkers should be aware of dietary restrictions to prevent accidental exposures. It's also essential for individuals to have a support system to lean on, as living with food restrictions can be challenging and emotionally taxing. In recent years, food manufacturers, restaurants, and foodservice providers have become more aware of the need to accommodate food allergies and sensitivities. Many establishments now offer allergen-friendly menus, gluten-free options, and clearly labeled allergen information. However, individuals with food allergies and sensitivities should still exercise caution and communicate their needs when dining out. Food allergies and sensitivities can impact not only dietary choices but also social and emotional well-being. Feelings of frustration, isolation, or anxiety can arise when navigating a world filled with food options that may be harmful. Seeking support from healthcare professionals, support groups, or mental health counselors can help individuals manage the emotional challenges associated with dietary restrictions.

Managing allergies and sensitivities in your diet requires a combination of vigilance, education, and support. For those with food allergies, strict avoidance of allergenic foods and carrying epinephrine are essential safety measures. For individuals with food sensitivities, identifying trigger foods, avoiding them, and maintaining a balanced diet with the guidance of a registered dietitian are crucial steps. Communication with restaurant staff and hosts, as well as education of friends and family, helps create a safe and inclusive environment. While managing allergies and sensitivities can be challenging, a proactive and informed approach can lead to a fulfilling and health-conscious lifestyle.

Chapter 7
The Joy of Cooking

Healthy Cooking Techniques

Healthy cooking techniques are the cornerstone of preparing nutritious and delicious meals that contribute to overall well-being. These techniques focus on optimizing nutrient retention while minimizing the use of unhealthy ingredients, such as excessive fats, sugars, and sodium. Learning and incorporating these techniques into your culinary repertoire can help you make healthier choices in the kitchen and enjoy nourishing meals. One fundamental healthy cooking technique is steaming. Steaming involves cooking food by exposing it to steam from boiling water. It's a gentle and effective method that helps preserve the natural colors, flavors, and nutrients in food. Vegetables, fish, and poultry are excellent candidates for steaming. Steamed vegetables maintain their vibrant colors and crisp textures, making them appealing and nutritious additions to any meal. Another key technique is sautéing, which involves cooking food in a small amount of oil or cooking spray over high heat in a shallow pan. Sautéing allows for quick cooking and browning of foods while preserving their natural flavors. It's important to use healthy cooking oils like olive oil or canola oil and avoid excessive amounts to keep the dish light and nutritious. Vegetables, lean proteins, and whole grains can all benefit from sautéing.

Grilling is a popular cooking technique that imparts a smoky and savory flavor to food. Grilling involves cooking food over an open flame or on a grill pan. While it's often associated with meats, grilling can be a healthy option for vegetables and fruits as well. To enhance the nutritional value of grilled dishes, marinate meats and vegetables in flavorful, healthy marinades made from herbs, spices, and a small amount of oil. Roasting is a versatile technique that is particularly well-suited for bringing out the natural sweetness and depth of flavor in a variety of ingredients. Whether you're roasting vegetables, chicken, or even fruits, this method involves cooking food in the oven at a moderate to high temperature. To keep roasted dishes healthy, use minimal oil, and consider adding herbs, spices, and citrus zest for flavor instead of salt and added fats. Poaching is a gentle cooking technique that involves submerging food, such as chicken, fish, or eggs, in simmering liquid, typically water or broth. Poaching helps food retain moisture and flavor without adding unnecessary fats. It's a great option for those looking to reduce their fat intake while enjoying tender and flavorful dishes. Poached chicken, for example, can be shredded and used in salads or sandwiches. Baking is a widely used cooking method for both sweet and savory dishes. It involves cooking food in an oven using dry heat. Baking can be a healthy technique when preparing dishes like whole-grain bread, baked fish, or vegetable casseroles. To maintain the nutritional value of baked goods, use whole grains, reduce added sugars, and incorporate fruits or vegetables for added moisture and flavor. Stir-frying is a quick and flavorful cooking technique originating from Asian cuisine. It involves cooking small, bite-sized pieces of food, such as vegetables and lean proteins, in a hot wok or skillet with a small amount of oil. Stir-frying preserves the vibrant colors and textures of ingredients while imparting a delicious umami flavor. To make stir-fries healthier, use lean meats or plant-based proteins and load up on colorful vegetables. Boiling is a straightforward cooking method that involves immersing food in boiling water until it is fully cooked. While boiling can lead to nutrient loss due to the leaching of water-soluble vitamins, it is still a practical way to prepare foods like pasta, rice, and certain vegetables. To retain nutrients, consider using the cooking water as a base for soups or sauces, or opt for whole grains and minimal cooking time. Blanching is a brief cooking method that involves immersing food in boiling water for a short period and then immediately transferring it to ice-cold water to stop the cooking process. Blanching is often used to preserve the color and texture of vegetables and fruits before freezing or further cooking. This technique can help retain nutrients and enhance the appearance of dishes. To enhance the nutritional profile of your meals, consider incorporating various herbs and spices. These natural flavor enhancers can add depth and complexity to dishes without the need for excess salt, sugar, or unhealthy fats. Experiment with a wide range of herbs like basil, thyme, and cilantro, as well as spices such as cumin, paprika, and turmeric. In addition to cooking techniques, portion control plays a vital role in maintaining a healthy diet. Be mindful of portion sizes to avoid overeating, which can lead to excess calorie intake. Using smaller plates and bowls can help control portion sizes and encourage mindful eating. It's important to remember that healthy cooking techniques are only part of the equation for maintaining a balanced diet. The selection of ingredients also matters significantly. Incorporate a variety of fruits, vegetables, whole grains, lean proteins, and healthy fats into your meals to ensure a diverse and nutrient-rich diet. Mastering healthy cooking techniques is essential for preparing nutritious and enjoyable meals. These techniques, including steaming, sautéing, grilling, roasting, poaching, baking, stir-frying, boiling, and blanching, allow you to create dishes that retain their natural flavors and nutrients while minimizing the use of unhealthy fats, sugars, and sodium. Alongside these techniques, the use of herbs and spices can elevate the taste of your dishes without relying on excessive salt or unhealthy flavor enhancers. Portion control and ingredient selection also play pivotal roles in maintaining a well-balanced diet. By incorporating these practices into your cooking routine, you can enjoy delicious, health-conscious meals that contribute to your overall well-being.

Recipes for Nutrient-Packed Meals

Creating recipes for nutrient-packed meals is a delicious and fulfilling way to ensure that your diet is rich in essential vitamins, minerals, and other beneficial compounds. Nutrient-dense meals are those that provide a high concentration of nutrients relative to their calorie content, making them an excellent choice for maintaining overall health and well-being. These meals are typically composed of whole foods, such as fruits, vegetables, lean proteins, whole grains, and healthy fats, which are packed with essential nutrients and antioxidants. One versatile and nutrient-packed meal option is the grain bowl. Grain bowls typically consist of a base of whole grains like quinoa, brown rice, or farro, which provide complex carbohydrates, fiber, and essential minerals. Top your grain bowl with an array of colorful vegetables, such as leafy greens, bell peppers, cherry tomatoes, and carrots, to maximize vitamins, minerals, and antioxidants. Add a source of lean protein, like grilled chicken, tofu, or chickpeas, to increase satiety and muscle support. Finally, drizzle with a flavorful vinaigrette made from heart-healthy olive oil, vinegar, and herbs for added taste

without excessive calories. Salads are another excellent way to create nutrient-packed meals. Start with a bed of leafy greens, such as spinach, kale, or arugula, to provide a wealth of vitamins, minerals, and fiber. Add a variety of colorful vegetables, such as cucumbers, red onions, and radishes, for added antioxidants and flavor. Incorporate lean proteins like grilled salmon, sliced turkey breast, or boiled eggs to boost protein intake. Finally, toss your salad with a homemade dressing made from olive oil, lemon juice, and a pinch of sea salt for a satisfying and nutritious meal. Soups and stews offer a comforting and nutrient-rich meal option. Begin by selecting a broth or base rich in flavor and low in sodium, such as vegetable or chicken broth. Add a variety of vegetables like carrots, celery, zucchini, and spinach to increase fiber and vitamins. Incorporate a lean source of protein, such as beans, lentils, or diced chicken breast, for a well-rounded meal. To enhance flavor without excessive salt, use herbs and spices like thyme, rosemary, cumin, and paprika. Enjoy your soup or stew with a side of whole-grain bread or a small serving of brown rice for added satiety and fiber.
For breakfast, consider nutrient-packed options like smoothie bowls. Blend a combination of fruits such as berries, bananas, and mangoes with Greek yogurt or plant-based yogurt for creaminess and probiotics. Add spinach or kale for an extra dose of vitamins and antioxidants. Top your smoothie bowl with a variety of toppings like nuts, seeds, granola, and fresh fruit for texture, crunch, and added nutrients. This breakfast option is not only visually appealing but also provides a range of vitamins, minerals, fiber, and healthy fats to start your day on the right foot. Another nutrient-packed breakfast idea is overnight oats. Combine rolled oats with your choice of milk, whether it's dairy, almond, soy, or coconut milk, and let the mixture soak overnight in the refrigerator. Add flavor and nutrients with ingredients like chia seeds, sliced almonds, and dried fruits. Top your oats with fresh berries, a drizzle of honey, and a sprinkle of cinnamon for a delicious and nutritious breakfast that provides fiber, vitamins, and minerals.
When it comes to nutrient-packed meals, it's important to be mindful of portion sizes. Even though these meals are rich in nutrients, consuming excessive calories can still lead to weight

gain. Pay attention to portion control, and consider using smaller plates and bowls to help regulate serving sizes. Recipes for nutrient-packed meals are essential for maintaining a healthy and

balanced diet. These meals are composed of whole foods that provide a high concentration of vitamins, minerals, and antioxidants relative to their calorie content. Grain bowls, salads, soups, smoothie bowls, and overnight oats are versatile meal options that offer a wide range of nutrients and flavors. By incorporating a variety of colorful fruits and vegetables, lean proteins, whole grains, and healthy fats into your meals, you can create nutrient-dense dishes that support overall well-being. Additionally, paying attention to portion sizes is crucial to ensure that you're not overindulging in calories while enjoying these nutritious meals.

Cooking with Love and Intention

Cooking with love and intention is a practice that goes beyond the mechanics of preparing food; it's about infusing your culinary creations with care, mindfulness, and a genuine appreciation for the nourishment and pleasure that food brings. When you cook with love and intention, you not only enhance the flavors of your dishes but also create a deeper connection to the food you prepare and the people you share it with. At the heart of cooking with love and intention is mindfulness. Mindfulness in cooking involves being fully present in the moment, focusing your attention on the task at hand, and appreciating each ingredient's unique qualities. When you approach cooking with mindfulness, you're less likely to rush through the process or multitask while preparing meals. Instead, you savor the sensory experience of cooking—feeling the textures, inhaling the aromas, and tasting as you go along. One of the essential aspects of mindful cooking is choosing high-quality ingredients. Pay attention to the source and quality of your ingredients, whether it's locally grown produce, sustainably sourced seafood, or organic grains. Knowing where your food comes from and how it was produced allows you to make informed choices that align with your values and contribute to a more sustainable and ethical food system. Another crucial element of cooking with love and intention is gratitude. Cultivate a sense of gratitude for the food you have access to and the ability to prepare it. Reflect on the journey of each ingredient, from the soil or sea to

your kitchen, and acknowledge the effort and care that went into producing and distributing it. Gratitude can enhance your connection to food and deepen your appreciation for the nourishment it provides. When you cook with love and intention, you prioritize the act of cooking as an act of self-care and nourishment. It's an opportunity to nurture your body and soul, to take a break from the demands of daily life, and to reconnect with your inner self. Cooking becomes a form of meditation, a way to de-stress, and a creative outlet for self-expression. Preparing meals intentionally allows you to be more attuned to your own needs and preferences, leading to healthier and more satisfying eating habits. Sharing food prepared with love and intention is a powerful way to foster connections with others. Whether you're cooking for family, friends, or yourself, the act of sharing a meal creates a sense of community and strengthens relationships. Cooking for loved ones can be an expression of care and affection, a way to celebrate milestones, and an opportunity to bond over shared experiences. Even when dining alone, cooking with love can be a form of self-love, nourishing not only your body but also your soul. Incorporating mindfulness and intention into your cooking can also lead to healthier and more balanced meals. When you pay close attention to the flavors, textures, and aromas of your food, you're more likely to make balanced and nutritious choices. You become attuned to your body's hunger and fullness cues, which can help prevent overeating and promote mindful eating. Additionally, cooking with intention allows you to experiment with new ingredients and flavors, expanding your culinary repertoire and making healthy eating more enjoyable. To practice cooking with love and intention, consider setting aside dedicated time for meal preparation, free from distractions and rushed schedules. Create a peaceful and inviting cooking environment, with soothing music, soft lighting, and a clutter-free workspace. Take a moment to set an intention for your meal, whether it's to nourish your body, express gratitude, or simply enjoy the process. As you cook, focus on your senses, noticing the colors, textures, and scents that surround you. Cooking with love and intention doesn't require elaborate or time-consuming recipes. Even simple dishes can be transformed when prepared mindfully and with care. It's about infusing your energy and presence into every step of the cooking process, from chopping vegetables to plating the final dish. When you approach cooking in this way, you'll find that even the most basic ingredients can become a source of joy and inspiration.Cooking with love and intention is a practice that elevates meal preparation from a mundane task to a mindful and enriching experience. It involves being fully present, choosing high-quality ingredients, cultivating gratitude, and using cooking as an act of self-care and connection. When you cook with love and intention, you not only create delicious and nourishing meals but also deepen your relationship with food and the people you share it with. This approach to cooking can lead to healthier eating habits, greater culinary creativity, and a profound sense of fulfillment in the kitchen.

Chapter 8
Dining Out and Social Eating

Making Healthy Choices at Restaurants

Making healthy choices at restaurants can be challenging, especially when faced with enticing menus full of delicious, but often calorie-laden, options. However, it is entirely possible to dine out while prioritizing your health and nutritional goals. Doing so requires a combination of mindful decision-making, menu navigation, and understanding key factors that influence the nutritional value of restaurant dishes. One of the most effective strategies for making healthy choices at restaurants is to plan ahead. Before dining out, take a moment to review the restaurant's menu online if available. This allows you to assess the options and identify dishes that align with your dietary preferences and nutritional goals. Look for menu items that feature lean proteins, plenty of vegetables, and whole grains. Avoid dishes described as "fried," "battered," "crispy," or "creamy," as these often indicate higher calorie and fat content. When you arrive at the restaurant, resist the temptation to make impulsive decisions based on hunger. Consider having a small, healthy snack before heading out to curb your appetite, so you're less likely to overindulge on bread or high-calorie appetizers while waiting for your meal. Additionally, try to stay hydrated with water or herbal tea, as thirst can sometimes be mistaken for hunger. When it comes to ordering, don't be afraid to customize your meal to suit your preferences and dietary needs. Many restaurants are accommodating and willing to make modifications to dishes. For example, you can request that your dish be prepared with less oil, butter, or salt. You can also ask for sauces, dressings, or cheese to be served on the side, allowing you to control the amount you use. Portion control is a critical aspect of healthy dining at restaurants. Keep in mind that restaurant portions are often larger than what you might typically serve yourself at home. Consider sharing an entrée with a dining partner or ask for a to-go container at the beginning of the meal to portion out half and save it for later. Alternatively, you can order appetizers or smaller plates, which tend to have more reasonable portion sizes. Pay attention to how dishes are prepared and cooked. Opt for grilled, baked, roasted, or steamed options over fried or deep-fried items. Dishes that are cooked with minimal added fats are generally lower in calories and healthier. Additionally, choose dishes that emphasize vegetables and lean proteins, such as grilled chicken or fish, as the main components. The choices you make regarding side dishes can significantly impact the overall nutritional content of your meal. Instead of fries or other fried sides, consider options like steamed vegetables, side salads, or whole grains. These sides are more likely to provide essential nutrients and fiber while keeping your meal balanced. Beware of the "hidden" ingredients in restaurant dishes. Many dishes may contain added sugars, unhealthy fats, or excessive sodium, which can contribute to less healthy choices. Keep an eye out for keywords on the menu that may indicate these hidden elements. For example, dishes described as "glazed," "smothered," or "sautéed in butter" are more likely to be higher in added sugars and unhealthy fats. Dining out often involves a social aspect, and while enjoying your meal, it's essential to engage in mindful eating. Focus on savoring each bite, appreciating the flavors, textures, and aromas of your food. Eat slowly and pay attention to your body's hunger and fullness cues. This mindful approach to dining can help prevent overeating and promote a greater sense of satisfaction with your meal. It's worth noting that some restaurants now offer nutrition information on their menus or websites, making it easier for patrons to make informed choices. When available, review this information to assess the calorie, fat, and sodium content of different dishes. Be cautious of portion sizes and make adjustments to suit your nutritional needs. In situations where nutrition information is not readily available, don't hesitate to ask your server for guidance. They can often provide insights into healthier menu options, suggest substitutions, and answer questions about ingredients or preparation methods. Restaurants are becoming increasingly aware of customers' dietary preferences and are often willing to accommodate special requests. Another aspect to consider is alcohol consumption. Alcoholic beverages, such as cocktails, wine, and beer, can contribute a significant number of calories to your meal. If you choose to drink alcohol, do so in moderation and be aware of the calorie content of your chosen beverages. Opt for lighter options like wine, spirits with low-calorie mixers, or simply enjoy water or unsweetened beverages with your meal. Lastly, remember that indulging occasionally is perfectly acceptable and can be a part of a balanced approach to dining out. If there's a dish you're particularly excited about, go ahead and enjoy it. The key is to find a balance between making healthy choices most of the time and allowing yourself occasional treats without guilt. In summary, making healthy choices at restaurants is entirely achievable with a combination of planning, mindfulness, and informed decision-making. Consider reviewing the menu in advance, customize your order to align with your dietary needs, control portion sizes, opt for healthier cooking methods, and be mindful of hidden ingredients. Engage in mindful eating, pay attention to your body's cues, and don't hesitate to ask for assistance from restaurant staff when needed. With these strategies in mind, you can dine out while maintaining your nutritional goals and overall health.

Navigating Social Situations

Navigating social situations is a fundamental aspect of our daily lives, and this holds true even within the context of the book "FOOD RELATIONSHIP - A Love Affair with Wellness." While the book primarily focuses on the relationship between individuals and their food choices, it indirectly addresses the importance of navigating social situations that revolve around food, nutrition, and well-being.

Effective communication is a central theme when it comes to discussing food choices and preferences with others. In social settings, whether it's a family dinner, a meal with friends, or a workplace lunch, people often have diverse opinions about food. These situations may lead to conversations about dietary restrictions, preferences, or ethical choices like vegetarianism or veganism. Navigating these discussions requires open, empathetic communication to foster understanding and respect for one another's choices. Empathy also plays a crucial role when considering social situations related to food. People have varied backgrounds, experiences, and reasons for their food choices. Some may have specific dietary requirements due to allergies or health conditions, while others may follow diets based on personal beliefs or ethical considerations. Understanding and empathizing with these differences can lead to more inclusive and harmonious social interactions, where everyone feels heard and respected.

Cultural awareness is another important aspect within social situations involving food. Food is deeply tied to culture, and individuals from diverse backgrounds may have unique culinary traditions and practices. Being aware of and respecting these cultural differences enhances our ability to navigate social gatherings respectfully. It also allows us to appreciate the richness of diverse cuisines and broaden our culinary horizons. Emotional intelligence, a theme woven throughout the book, is closely related to navigating social situations. Emotional intelligence involves recognizing, understanding, and managing emotions, both in ourselves and in others. When it comes to food and social interactions, emotional intelligence enables us to perceive the emotional cues of those around us. It helps us respond empathetically to someone who may be struggling with their relationship with food, offering support and understanding rather than judgment. Assertiveness in social situations can be particularly important. The book encourages individuals to make informed, health-conscious food choices. In social settings where indulgent or unhealthy food options may be abundant, being assertive can help individuals stay true to their dietary goals without feeling pressured to make choices that don't align with their well-being. Assertiveness allows people to express their preferences and boundaries while respecting the choices of others. Conflict resolution, often a part of social situations involving food, is a skill that the book indirectly addresses. Conflicts may arise when individuals have differing opinions on what constitutes a healthy diet or when someone feels judged for their food choices. Resolving these conflicts constructively requires active listening, empathy, and a focus on finding common ground. The principles of conflict resolution outlined in the book can be applied to navigate such situations effectively. Furthermore, "FOOD RELATIONSHIP - A Love Affair with Wellness" emphasizes the importance of mindful eating, which can be practiced not only in solitary moments but also in social settings. When dining with others, mindful eating involves being fully present during the meal, savoring each bite, and engaging in meaningful conversations rather than rushing through the experience. This approach can enhance social interactions around food, making meals more enjoyable and fostering a deeper connection with both the food and the people sharing it.

Respect for personal boundaries is paramount in any social situation, including those involving food. It's crucial to recognize and honor the dietary restrictions, allergies, or preferences of others. Respecting these boundaries fosters trust and consideration within the group, ensuring that everyone can enjoy the meal without worry or discomfort. Networking, a concept often associated with professional contexts, can also apply to social situations involving food. Individuals who share a common interest in health-conscious eating or specific dietary choices can connect and support each other in their journeys. Sharing recipes, meal ideas, and experiences can create a sense of community and offer valuable resources for maintaining a positive relationship with food. Lastly, building and maintaining trust is essential in all social situations, especially when it comes to food and nutrition. Trust is the foundation of any healthy relationship, and this extends to the choices individuals make regarding their diets. Trustworthy individuals are reliable in their commitments to making health-conscious food choices, and they respect the choices of others without judgment. This trust-building approach contributes to harmonious social interactions around food. Navigating social situations involves effective communication, empathy, cultural awareness, emotional intelligence, assertiveness, conflict resolution, mindful eating, respect for personal boundaries, networking, and trust-building. These skills are essential for fostering positive and meaningful interactions with others in various social settings where food and nutrition are central themes. By applying these principles, individuals can create an environment that supports their well-being while also respecting the diverse choices and preferences of those they interact with.

Traveling and Eating Well

Traveling and eating well are not mutually exclusive; in fact, they can complement each other beautifully. Traveling presents unique opportunities to explore diverse cuisines, savor new flavors, and immerse oneself in local culinary traditions. However, it can also pose challenges to maintaining a balanced and health-conscious diet. To strike a harmonious balance between culinary adventure and well-being while on the road, it's essential to adopt a mindful and informed approach to eating during travel. One of the key principles of eating well while traveling is preparation. Before embarking on your journey, take some time to research the culinary landscape of your destination. Seek out local dishes that are both delicious and nutritious. Explore the availability of fresh fruits, vegetables, and whole grains. Familiarize yourself with the eating habits and portion sizes of the local culture. This knowledge will empower you to make informed food choices and adapt your preferences to the available options. When traveling, staying hydrated is essential for overall well-being. Carry a reusable water bottle to ensure you have access to clean drinking water throughout your journey. Dehydration can lead to fatigue and discomfort, so prioritize hydration to stay energized and ready to explore. While indulging in local cuisine is a highlight of travel, it's essential to practice moderation. Portion control can be challenging when presented with new and exciting dishes, but overeating can lead to discomfort and unwanted weight gain. One strategy is to share meals with travel companions to sample a variety of dishes without consuming excessive calories. Balancing indulgent meals with lighter options is another effective approach. Seek out restaurants or eateries that offer salads, grilled or steamed dishes, and fresh seafood or lean protein options. These choices can help you maintain a balanced diet while still enjoying the local food culture. Moreover, explore local markets and street vendors to discover fresh and nutritious snacks. Fruits, nuts, and yogurt are often readily available and make for convenient and healthy on-the-go options. These snacks provide essential nutrients and keep you fueled for your travel adventures. Mindful eating, a concept emphasized throughout the book, is especially relevant when traveling. In the midst of new experiences and unfamiliar cuisines, it's easy to rush through meals or eat mindlessly. Instead, make an effort to savor each bite, appreciate the flavors, and engage all your senses. Mindful eating allows you to fully enjoy your meals and make more conscious choices. Consider the importance of balance during your travels. While it's tempting to indulge in local specialties, strive to maintain a balanced diet that includes a variety of food groups. Incorporate fruits and vegetables into your meals whenever possible to ensure you receive essential vitamins and minerals. Balance higher-calorie meals with lighter options to avoid overconsumption. Exploring local cuisine also presents an opportunity to expand your culinary horizons. Be open to trying new foods and flavors, even if they are outside your usual comfort zone. Experimenting with different dishes can be a memorable part of your travel experience. Embrace the adventure and appreciate the diversity of world cuisines. Furthermore, consider the timing of your meals while traveling. Irregular eating patterns can disrupt your digestive system and energy levels. Strive for a consistent meal schedule that aligns with your body's natural rhythms. Avoid skipping meals, as this can lead to overeating later in the day. Instead, plan regular, balanced meals to keep your energy steady. Local food tours and cooking classes can be a delightful way to engage with the culinary culture of your destination. These experiences offer insights into traditional cooking techniques, local ingredients, and the stories behind beloved dishes. Engaging with local food experts and fellow travelers can enhance your appreciation for regional cuisine. Additionally, be mindful of food safety while traveling. In some regions, tap water may not be safe to drink, and certain foods may pose health risks. Prioritize safe food handling and hygiene practices to avoid foodborne illnesses. Familiarize yourself with local guidelines and recommendations, such as avoiding street food that may not be prepared under sanitary conditions. When dining out, consider asking your server about ingredient options and preparation methods. If you have dietary restrictions or allergies, communicate these clearly to ensure your safety and enjoyment. Many restaurants are accommodating and willing to make adjustments to accommodate your needs. Snacking can be an enjoyable part of travel, but choose snacks wisely. Opt for nutritious options like fresh fruit, nuts, or yogurt instead of heavily processed, high-calorie snacks. These healthier choices can provide sustained energy and keep you feeling your best during your adventures. In summary, traveling and eating well are not only compatible but can enhance your overall travel experience. Preparation, hydration, portion control, moderation, balance, mindful eating, and openness to new flavors are key principles to keep in mind. While indulging in local cuisine is a highlight of travel, maintaining a balanced diet and food safety practices are equally important. Embrace culinary exploration, engage with the local food culture, and savor each bite to create lasting memories and savor the journey.

Chapter 9

Sustainable Eating

The Environmental Impact of Food Choices

The environmental impact of food choices is a complex and critical issue that affects the health of our planet and future generations. It encompasses various aspects of food production, distribution, and consumption, all of which contribute to the sustainability of our global food system. Understanding these impacts and making informed choices about what we eat can play a significant role in mitigating environmental damage. One of the most substantial environmental impacts of food choices is related to greenhouse gas emissions. The production of animal-based foods, such as beef, pork, and dairy, is a major contributor to greenhouse gas emissions, particularly methane and nitrous oxide. Livestock farming requires extensive resources, including land, water, and feed, which, in turn, leads to deforestation, habitat destruction, and water pollution. Adopting a more plant-based diet and reducing meat consumption can substantially lower greenhouse gas emissions associated with food production. The agricultural sector is a major consumer of freshwater resources, and the way we produce and consume food has a significant impact on water scarcity. Crop irrigation, livestock farming, and food processing all demand substantial amounts of water. Unsustainable water use in agriculture can lead to over-extraction of water from rivers and aquifers, causing ecological imbalances and threatening the availability of freshwater for future generations. Choosing foods that are less water-intensive, such as vegetables and grains, can help reduce the environmental strain on water resources. Food waste is a pressing environmental concern. Globally, a substantial portion of food produced is wasted at various stages of the supply chain, from production and distribution to consumption. Food waste not only squanders valuable resources like water, energy, and land but also generates greenhouse gas emissions as the discarded food decomposes in landfills. Reducing food waste at both the individual and institutional levels can significantly contribute to minimizing the environmental impact of our food choices. Monoculture farming practices, where large areas of land are dedicated to growing a single crop, can lead to soil degradation, loss of biodiversity, and increased vulnerability to pests and diseases. Such practices often rely heavily on chemical pesticides and fertilizers, which can harm ecosystems, contaminate water sources, and contribute to the decline of pollinators like bees. Choosing foods that are sustainably and diversely grown, such as organic or regeneratively farmed produce, can help mitigate these negative environmental effects. The seafood industry also poses significant environmental challenges. Overfishing, illegal fishing, and bycatch (the unintentional capture of non-target species) can harm marine ecosystems and deplete fish populations. Unsustainable fishing practices not only threaten food security but also disrupt marine ecosystems and contribute to habitat destruction. Opting for sustainably sourced seafood, as certified by organizations like the Marine Stewardship Council (MSC) or the Aquaculture Stewardship Council (ASC), can support responsible fishing practices and promote marine conservation. Genetically modified organisms (GMOs) are a contentious issue in the realm of food choices and environmental impact. While proponents argue that GMOs can increase crop yields and reduce the need for chemical pesticides, critics express concerns about their long-term effects on ecosystems and biodiversity. The debate around GMOs highlights the importance of informed choices and transparency in our food system. Consumers can choose to support or avoid GMOs based on their own values and concerns. Transportation and food miles are additional factors to consider. The distance that food travels from its place of production to the consumer, known as food miles, can have implications for greenhouse gas emissions and energy consumption. Choosing locally sourced foods, when possible, can reduce the environmental footprint associated with transportation. Supporting farmers' markets, community-supported agriculture (CSA), and seasonal produce can promote local food systems and reduce the need for long-distance transportation. The packaging and processing of food products also contribute to their environmental impact. Excessive packaging, especially single-use plastics, can generate a significant amount of waste and pollution.

Opting for products with minimal or recyclable packaging can help mitigate this issue. Additionally, choosing minimally processed foods can reduce the energy and resources required for food processing. The practice of buying and consuming in-season foods can have environmental benefits. Seasonal foods are often more readily available and require fewer resources for production and transportation. Embracing seasonal eating can support local agriculture, reduce the environmental footprint of your food choices, and connect you with the rhythms of nature.

Finally, food choices can have indirect effects on land use and conservation efforts. For example, the demand for palm oil, a common ingredient in processed foods, has driven deforestation in tropical regions, threatening wildlife habitats and increasing carbon emissions. Becoming more aware of the ingredients in the products we consume and choosing those that are sourced sustainably can contribute to conservation efforts and protect precious ecosystems.

The environmental impact of food choices is a multifaceted issue that encompasses various aspects of food production, distribution, and consumption. Understanding these impacts and making informed choices about what we eat is essential for reducing our carbon footprint, conserving natural resources, and promoting a more sustainable and resilient food system. By considering factors such as greenhouse gas emissions, water use, food waste, sustainable sourcing, transportation, packaging, and the indirect consequences of our food choices, we can play a vital role in preserving the health of our planet for future generations.

Supporting Local and Sustainable Food Systems

Supporting local and sustainable food systems is a powerful way to promote environmental sustainability, strengthen local economies, and improve the overall quality of our food. These choices have far-reaching impacts, touching on everything from reducing greenhouse gas emissions to enhancing community resilience. Embracing local and sustainable food systems involves a holistic approach that encompasses various elements of our food supply chain. Local food systems prioritize sourcing food from nearby producers, reducing the distance between the farm and the consumer. This approach offers numerous benefits, including a reduced carbon footprint due to shorter transportation distances. It also supports local farmers and strengthens regional food economies. By choosing to buy locally grown produce and products, consumers can help create a more resilient and vibrant food system. Community-supported agriculture (CSA) programs are a prime example of local food systems in action. These programs allow consumers to purchase shares of a local farm's harvest, thereby establishing a direct connection between producers and consumers. CSA members receive regular deliveries of fresh, seasonal produce, and in return, they provide financial support to local farmers, ensuring a stable income. Farmers' markets are another cornerstone of local food systems. These markets bring together local farmers and artisans to sell their products directly to consumers. Shoppers can access fresh, locally grown produce, meat, dairy, and artisanal goods while enjoying a sense of community and connection with the people who produce their food. Sustainable food systems prioritize environmentally responsible and ethical practices throughout the food supply chain. Sustainable agriculture aims to minimize negative environmental impacts, conserve natural resources, and protect biodiversity. It also promotes fair labor practices and equitable treatment of workers in the food industry. Supporting sustainable food systems means making choices that align with these principles. One significant aspect of sustainability is organic farming, which avoids synthetic pesticides and fertilizers, focusing instead on natural and environmentally friendly methods. Organic farming helps preserve soil health, reduce water pollution, and protect ecosystems from the adverse effects of chemical pesticides. Choosing organic products supports these practices and encourages the growth of sustainable agriculture. Regenerative agriculture is an emerging concept within sustainable food systems that goes beyond simply minimizing harm to the environment. It aims to actively restore ecosystems and enhance soil health. By supporting regenerative agriculture, consumers promote practices that can sequester carbon, improve water retention, and revitalize landscapes. Another essential component of sustainable food systems is responsible fisheries and aquaculture. Unsustainable fishing practices can deplete fish populations and harm marine ecosystems. By choosing sustainably sourced seafood, consumers help protect oceans and promote responsible fishing practices. Certifications such as the Marine Stewardship Council (MSC) and the Aquaculture Stewardship Council (ASC) guide consumers toward responsible seafood choices. Supporting local and sustainable food systems also involves reducing food waste. Globally, a substantial amount of food is wasted at various stages of the supply chain, from production to consumption. Consumers can help reduce food waste by buying only what they need, properly storing food to extend its shelf life, and finding creative ways to use leftovers. Additionally, supporting initiatives that rescue and redistribute surplus food to those in need can address food waste while combating hunger. Urban agriculture is another vital aspect of sustainable food systems. It involves growing food in urban environments, often in community gardens or on rooftops. Urban agriculture enhances food security, reduces the carbon footprint of food transportation, and connects city dwellers with the source of their food. Supporting urban agriculture initiatives can promote sustainable, localized food production. Community food co-ops and food hubs are essential components of local and sustainable food systems. These community-driven organizations bring together local producers and consumers to provide access to fresh, locally sourced foods. Co-ops often emphasize fair pricing for both producers and consumers, making high-quality, sustainably produced food accessible to a broader range of people. Education plays a significant role in supporting local and sustainable food systems. Raising awareness about the environmental and social impacts of food choices can inspire consumers to make more informed decisions. Educational programs, workshops, and initiatives that teach people about sustainable agriculture, food preservation, and cooking skills can empower individuals to make positive changes in their food consumption habits. Institutional and policy support is crucial for scaling up local and sustainable food systems. Governments, businesses, and organizations can play a pivotal role in creating an environment that supports sustainable agriculture, responsible food production, and equitable access to healthy foods. Policies that incentivize sustainable farming practices, promote local sourcing in public institutions, and regulate food labeling can help drive positive change in the food system.

Supporting local and sustainable food systems also fosters food sovereignty, which empowers communities to control their own food production and distribution. This approach prioritizes local food systems and community decision-making over centralized corporate control. It strengthens communities' ability to determine their food choices, promote cultural diversity in diets, and protect their local environments. Overall, embracing local and sustainable food systems involves a conscious and informed approach to our food choices. It means seeking out locally grown and produced foods, supporting sustainable agriculture, reducing food waste, and promoting equitable access to healthy foods. These choices have the power to transform our food system, making it more environmentally responsible, socially just, and resilient in the face of global challenges. By aligning our values and preferences with local and sustainable food options, we can contribute to a more sustainable and equitable future for our food system and the planet.

Reducing Food Waste

Reducing food waste is a pressing global challenge that has significant economic, environmental, and social implications. Every year, an estimated one-third of all food produced for human consumption is lost or wasted, representing a staggering 1.3 billion tons of food. This waste occurs throughout the entire food supply chain, from production and distribution to retail and consumer levels. Addressing food waste requires a concerted effort from individuals, businesses, and governments to minimize the inefficiencies in our food system.

At the consumer level, awareness and responsible food management play a pivotal role in reducing waste. One of the primary ways consumers can combat food waste is by practicing mindful shopping and meal planning. This involves making grocery lists, purchasing only what is needed, and avoiding impulse buys. It's crucial to take stock of the ingredients already on hand and plan meals that incorporate items that are nearing their expiration dates. By doing so, consumers can significantly reduce the amount of food that ends up being discarded.

Proper food storage is another essential component of reducing waste. Ensuring that perishable items are stored at the correct temperature and in suitable conditions can extend their shelf life. This includes using airtight containers, refrigerating items promptly, and keeping an organized pantry to avoid items getting lost and forgotten. Understanding food labels, such as "best before" and "use by" dates, can also help consumers make informed decisions about the safety and freshness of their food. Creative cooking and repurposing leftovers are effective strategies to minimize waste. Consumers can transform surplus ingredients or meals into new dishes or freeze them for later use. For example, leftover vegetables can be turned into soups or stir-fries, and stale bread can be used for breadcrumbs or croutons. Reducing plate waste by serving appropriate portion sizes is equally important. It's better to have a second helping than to discard food that has been served but not consumed. In addition to individual actions, businesses play a significant role in addressing food waste. Food retailers and restaurants can implement practices that minimize waste, such as optimizing inventory management, donating surplus food to charitable organizations, and incorporating imperfect or surplus produce into their menus. The "ugly food" movement, which embraces imperfect-looking fruits and vegetables, is gaining momentum as a way to reduce waste at the production and retail levels. Technological innovations, such as smart refrigerators and food tracking apps, can help consumers and businesses manage food inventory more effectively. These tools can provide real-time information on food freshness, suggest recipes based on available ingredients, and send reminders about items that need to be used before they spoil. Another critical aspect of reducing food waste is redirecting surplus food to those in need. Food rescue organizations and food banks play a crucial role in redistributing surplus food to vulnerable populations. Businesses and individuals can support these organizations by donating excess food, volunteering their time, or contributing financially. This not only helps reduce waste but also addresses issues of food insecurity and hunger. Reducing food waste extends beyond individual actions and involves systemic changes within the food industry. One such change is a shift in consumer expectations regarding food aesthetics. Encouraging consumers to embrace "imperfect" produce and products can reduce the pressure on farmers and manufacturers to discard perfectly edible items that do not meet strict cosmetic standards. Governments and policymakers also have a role to play in reducing food waste. Regulations and incentives can encourage businesses to adopt waste reduction practices, such as tax incentives for food donations or regulations that prevent supermarkets from discarding edible food. Public awareness campaigns can educate consumers about the impacts of food waste and provide practical tips for reducing it. Furthermore, food waste is closely tied to the issue of overproduction in agriculture. Farmers often overproduce food to meet market demands, leading to a surplus that is discarded. Shifting to more sustainable and efficient agricultural practices, such as precision farming and reducing monoculture farming, can help align production with actual needs and reduce the overall volume of food waste.

Food waste is not solely an issue of wasted resources; it also has significant environmental consequences. When food ends up in landfills, it decomposes and produces methane, a potent greenhouse gas that contributes to climate change. Reducing food waste can significantly reduce methane emissions and mitigate the environmental impact of our food system.

Reducing food waste is a multifaceted challenge that requires collective action from individuals, businesses, and governments. Mindful shopping, responsible food management, proper storage, creative cooking, and supporting food rescue organizations are essential steps individuals can take. Businesses can optimize inventory management, repurpose surplus food, and embrace the imperfect food movement. Governments can enact policies and regulations that incentivize waste reduction and support food redistribution efforts. Ultimately, addressing food waste is not only about saving money and resources but also about preserving the environment and ensuring that everyone has access to the nourishment they need. By taking action at multiple levels of the food system, we can work towards a more sustainable and equitable future.

Chapter 10
Maintaining a Healthy Relationship with Food

The Long-Term Approach to Wellness

A long-term approach to wellness is a holistic and sustainable way of living that prioritizes health, both physical and mental, over the course of one's lifetime. It involves adopting habits and practices that promote well-being, prevent illness, and enhance the overall quality of life. This approach recognizes that health is not just the absence of disease but a state of optimal physical, mental, and emotional functioning. At the core of a long-term approach to wellness is the idea of prevention. Instead of waiting for health issues to arise and then seeking treatment, individuals proactively engage in behaviors that reduce the risk of illness. This includes maintaining a balanced diet, engaging in regular physical activity, getting adequate sleep, and managing stress effectively. Preventive measures can significantly reduce the likelihood of chronic diseases such as heart disease, diabetes, and certain cancers. Physical fitness is a central pillar of long-term wellness. Engaging in regular exercise has a myriad of health benefits, including improved cardiovascular health, stronger bones and muscles, enhanced flexibility, and better weight management. Exercise also releases endorphins, which contribute to a positive mood and mental well-being. Long-term wellness includes finding physical activities that one enjoys and can sustain over a lifetime, whether it's walking, swimming, yoga, or other forms of exercise. Nutrition is another crucial element of long-term wellness. A balanced diet that includes a variety of nutrient-dense foods provides the body with essential vitamins, minerals, and energy. Whole grains, fruits, vegetables, lean proteins, and healthy fats form the foundation of a nutritious diet. Limiting the consumption of processed foods, sugary beverages, and excessive amounts of salt and sugar is essential for preventing chronic diseases and maintaining a healthy weight. Mental health is an integral component of long-term wellness. Practicing stress management techniques such as mindfulness, meditation, and relaxation exercises can reduce the harmful effects of chronic stress on both the body and mind. Developing resilience and coping skills can help individuals navigate life's challenges more effectively, leading to better mental health outcomes in the long run.The importance of sleep in long-term wellness cannot be overstated. Quality sleep is essential for physical and mental recovery, memory consolidation, and overall well-being. Chronic sleep deprivation is associated with a range of health issues, including obesity, diabetes, and mood disorders. Adopting good sleep hygiene practices, such as maintaining a consistent sleep schedule and creating a comfortable sleep environment, supports long-term health and vitality. Social connections and emotional well-being are key aspects of long-term wellness. Strong social support networks and meaningful relationships contribute to a sense of belonging and emotional resilience. Engaging in activities that bring joy and fulfillment, as well as seeking professional help when needed, are important for maintaining mental and emotional health over the long term. A long-term approach to wellness also includes regular health check-ups and screenings to detect and address potential health issues early. Preventive measures such as vaccinations and screenings for conditions like cancer and cardiovascular disease can increase the chances of successful treatment when problems are identified in their early stages. Avoiding harmful behaviors such as smoking, excessive alcohol consumption, and substance abuse is fundamental to long-term wellness. These behaviors are associated with a host of health problems, including addiction, respiratory illnesses, and increased risk of accidents. Long-term wellness encourages the adoption of healthier alternatives and provides support for those looking to break free from harmful habits. Furthermore, environmental awareness is a growing aspect of long-term wellness. Being mindful of the environmental impact of one's lifestyle choices, such as reducing waste, conserving energy, and supporting sustainable practices, aligns with a broader sense of well-being that extends beyond personal health. Recognizing the interdependence of human health and the health of the planet is crucial for long-term sustainability. A long-term approach to wellness recognizes that health is a dynamic and evolving process. It involves setting realistic goals, adapting to life's changes and challenges, and being patient with oneself. Wellness is not a destination but a lifelong journey that requires ongoing commitment and self-care. By prioritizing prevention, physical fitness, nutrition, mental health, sleep, social connections, regular check-ups, healthy behaviors, and environmental awareness, individuals can lay the foundation for a healthier and more fulfilling life that spans not just years, but decades. Ultimately, the pursuit of long-term wellness is an investment in a brighter and healthier future, both for individuals and for society as a whole.

Overcoming Setbacks and Challenges

This book offers invaluable guidance on the journey towards a healthier relationship with food and overall well-being. However, like any meaningful transformation, the path to wellness can be peppered with setbacks and challenges. It's essential to recognize these hurdles and develop strategies to overcome them, ensuring long-term success in embracing a healthier lifestyle. Setbacks in the pursuit of a healthier relationship with food can often stem from deeply ingrained habits and emotional connections to eating. Emotional eating, for instance, may resurface during times of stress, sadness, or even celebration, leading to overindulgence and feelings of guilt. Overcoming this challenge involves cultivating mindfulness around emotional triggers and developing healthier coping mechanisms.

Another common setback is falling back into old dietary patterns and cravings. The allure of highly processed, sugary, or fatty foods can be strong, particularly in moments of weakness or fatigue. This challenge underscores the importance of gradual dietary changes and finding healthier alternatives that still satisfy your taste buds. External influences, such as societal pressures or the availability of unhealthy foods, can also present obstacles. Peer pressure, advertising, and the convenience of fast food can all derail your progress towards a healthier diet. Overcoming these influences requires reinforcing your commitment to your well-being and making conscious choices that align with your health goals. Inconsistency in maintaining healthy habits can be a significant setback. Starting with enthusiasm but gradually losing motivation or giving in to procrastination can hinder progress. Establishing a routine and setting realistic, achievable goals can help maintain consistency and prevent setbacks due to lapses in self-discipline. Additionally, unrealistic expectations can be a significant challenge on the journey to wellness. Rapid weight loss or dramatic dietary changes may not be sustainable or healthy. Embracing gradual, sustainable changes, and understanding that progress may have its ups and downs can help navigate this challenge. Environmental factors, such as limited access to healthy food options or a lack of time for meal preparation, can also be hurdles. Strategies like meal planning, batch cooking, and seeking out local markets or healthy takeout options can help address these challenges and make healthier choices more accessible. Moreover, self-criticism and negative self-talk can contribute to setbacks. Feelings of guilt or shame after indulging in less healthy foods can create a cycle of unhealthy eating habits. Developing self-compassion, self-forgiveness, and a positive mindset is essential for overcoming these emotional hurdles.

Family and social dynamics can also present challenges. Loved ones may not fully understand or support your dietary choices, making it challenging to maintain a healthy eating pattern during social gatherings or family meals. Open communication, setting boundaries, and finding compromise can help navigate these situations without compromising your goals. Addressing setbacks and challenges in the pursuit of a healthier relationship with food requires resilience, self-awareness, and a willingness to adapt. Mindfulness techniques can help you become more attuned to your emotional triggers and eating habits. Additionally, seeking support from a therapist, counselor, or a support group can provide valuable guidance and motivation to overcome emotional and psychological challenges. Incorporating stress-reduction practices, such as meditation, yoga, or deep breathing exercises, can help manage emotional eating triggers and maintain a sense of balance. Building a robust support network of friends and family who understand and respect your goals can also provide invaluable encouragement during challenging times. Furthermore, embracing the concept of "progress, not perfection" can help reframe setbacks as opportunities for growth rather than failures. Acknowledging that it's normal to face obstacles on the path to wellness can reduce feelings of guilt and self-criticism.

Setbacks can be an integral part of the journey towards a healthier relationship with food and overall well-being. By recognizing these challenges, developing strategies to overcome them, and fostering self-compassion, individuals can navigate the ups and downs with resilience and determination. Ultimately, the setbacks can serve as valuable learning experiences that contribute to long-term success in loving the food that loves you back.

Cultivating Self-Compassion

Cultivating self-compassion is a fundamental aspect of the journey toward a healthier relationship with food. This practice revolves around treating oneself with the same kindness, understanding, and forgiveness that one would offer to a close friend or loved one. It is a powerful tool for transforming negative self-talk, overcoming setbacks, and fostering a positive and sustainable approach to eating and overall well-being. One key component of self-compassion is developing a non-judgmental attitude towards oneself. Often, individuals can be their harshest critics, especially when it comes to food choices and body image. Self-compassion encourages individuals to let go of self-criticism and replace it with self-acceptance. This means acknowledging that everyone makes mistakes, including dietary ones, and that these do not define one's worth or character. Self-compassion allows individuals to view their imperfections as part of being human rather than as failures. Another essential element of self-compassion is self-kindness. This involves treating oneself with the same level of warmth, care, and encouragement that one would offer to a friend facing similar challenges. When it comes to food and wellness, self-kindness means speaking to oneself in a gentle and supportive manner. Rather than berating oneself for overindulging or making less healthy choices, individuals practicing self-compassion might say, "It's okay; we all have off days. Let's refocus on making healthier choices moving forward." This shift in self-talk can significantly impact one's emotional well-being and ability to maintain positive habits. Moreover, self-compassion encourages individuals to recognize and validate their emotions and experiences. This includes acknowledging feelings of guilt, shame, or frustration related to food choices or body image. Instead of suppressing or denying these emotions, self-compassion involves giving them space and understanding. It's about recognizing that these feelings are natural responses to life's challenges and that one does not have to be perfect or always in control. Self-compassion also extends to the concept of common humanity, which reminds individuals that they are not alone in their struggles. Everyone faces challenges and setbacks when it comes to food and well-being. By recognizing that others share similar experiences, individuals can feel more connected and less isolated in their journeys. This sense of shared humanity can provide comfort and motivation to persevere through difficult times.

Self-compassion plays a crucial role in overcoming challenges and setbacks. It offers a nurturing and forgiving perspective on moments of overindulgence or veering off course from healthier eating habits. Instead of dwelling on perceived failures, individuals can approach these situations with understanding and self-kindness, allowing them to move forward with a renewed commitment to their well-being. Self-compassion can also address emotional eating, a common challenge on the path to a healthier relationship with food. Emotional eating often arises from using food as a coping mechanism for stress, sadness, or other emotions. Self-compassion encourages individuals to explore the underlying emotional triggers for such behaviors with curiosity and compassion. Rather than judging oneself for turning to food in moments of emotional distress, self-compassion can offer alternative ways to manage emotions, such as mindfulness, meditation, or seeking support from others. In addition to its role in individual well-being, self-compassion can positively impact interpersonal relationships. When individuals practice self-compassion, they tend to be more understanding and forgiving of others' imperfections and struggles. This can foster healthier and more supportive dynamics within families, friendships, and communities, promoting a culture of empathy and acceptance. Practicing self-compassion is not a one-size-fits-all endeavor. It requires self-awareness and an ongoing commitment to change negative self-talk and cultivate self-kindness. Techniques such as self-compassion journaling, where individuals write compassionate letters to themselves, or mindfulness practices that promote self-acceptance, can be valuable tools in this process. Furthermore, self-compassion is not about relinquishing personal responsibility or enabling unhealthy behaviors. Rather, it is about approaching wellness with a balanced perspective, recognizing that self-improvement is a journey with its ups and downs. It encourages individuals to learn from their experiences, celebrate their successes, and adapt to their challenges with kindness and resilience. Cultivating self-compassion is a transformative practice on the journey toward a healthier relationship with food and overall well-being. It involves treating oneself with kindness, letting go of self-judgment, acknowledging one's emotions, and recognizing our shared humanity. Self-compassion empowers individuals to overcome setbacks, embrace imperfections, and approach wellness with a balanced and nurturing mindset. By incorporating self-compassion into their lives, individuals can foster lasting positive change and create a more compassionate and accepting relationship with themselves and the food they choose to love.

Embracing a Lifelong Love for Food

Embracing a lifelong love for food is a journey that transcends the mere act of eating; it is a profound and enduring relationship that can enrich our lives in countless ways. Food is not just sustenance; it is a source of pleasure, nourishment, and connection. It has the power to shape our physical health, influence our emotional well-being, and foster a deep sense of community.

At the heart of this lifelong love affair with food is a profound respect for its role in our lives. Food is not the enemy, nor is it a mere source of calories to be counted and restricted. It is a source of vitality, energy, and the building blocks that our bodies need to thrive. When we view food through this lens of respect and appreciation, we can make choices that honor our bodies and support our well-being. Moreover, embracing a lifelong love for food means savoring each bite and relishing the sensory experience of eating. It involves engaging all our senses—taste, smell, sight, touch, and even sound—when we sit down to a meal. By savoring the flavors and textures of our food, we not only enhance our enjoyment but also cultivate mindfulness, which can lead to healthier eating habits. Part of this lifelong love is recognizing that food is intimately tied to our cultural and social identities. It is a means of connecting with our heritage, celebrating traditions, and forging bonds with family and friends. By embracing the foods of our culture and sharing meals with loved ones, we honor the rich tapestry of human culinary diversity and strengthen the bonds that nourish our souls. A critical aspect of lifelong love for food is nurturing a positive relationship with our bodies. Rather than succumbing to societal pressures to attain a specific body image, we focus on nourishing and caring for our bodies as they are. This involves rejecting diet culture and unrealistic beauty standards and instead listening to our bodies' signals of hunger and fullness. In this journey, we also discover the joy of cooking and preparing meals. Preparing our food allows us to connect with the ingredients, savor the creative process, and gain a deeper appreciation for the effort that goes into each dish. Cooking can become a form of self-expression and a way to explore new flavors and cuisines. Furthermore, lifelong love for food involves balance and moderation. It acknowledges that there is room for all foods in our lives, and no single food should be entirely off-limits. By practicing moderation and portion control, we can enjoy our favorite treats without guilt while ensuring that our overall diet is balanced and nutritious. As we traverse this lifelong love affair with food, we recognize the importance of nourishing not only our bodies but also our minds and souls. Food has the power to uplift our spirits, evoke cherished memories, and bring us comfort in times of need. By approaching our meals with gratitude and mindfulness, we can derive not only physical nourishment but also emotional and spiritual fulfillment. The journey toward a lifelong love for food is not without its challenges. We will encounter moments of temptation, emotional eating, and setbacks on our path. But these challenges, when approached with self-compassion and resilience, become opportunities for growth and learning. They remind us that our relationship with food is dynamic and ever-evolving. In conclusion, embracing a lifelong love for food is an exquisite journey of self-discovery, connection, and well-being. It is a journey that invites us to savor each moment, cherish our bodies, celebrate our culture, and find joy in the act of nourishing ourselves and others. It is a lifelong commitment to a relationship that sustains us physically, emotionally, and spiritually, enriching our lives in countless ways. As we continue on this path, let us remember that food, when approached with love and respect, has the power to love us back with vitality, health, and enduring happiness.

Conclusion

In conclusion, "FOOD RELATIONSHIP - A Love Affair with Wellness" has been a journey of self-discovery, empowerment, and transformation through the lens of mindful and balanced eating. This book has explored a wide array of topics, from the fundamentals of nutrition and the Plate Method to the intricacies of emotional eating and the mindful appreciation of food. It has offered practical steps, insightful reflections, and a wealth of knowledge to guide you on your path to a healthier and more fulfilling relationship with food. Throughout these pages, we've delved into the power of mindful eating, uncovering its ability to nourish not only our bodies but also our minds and spirits. We've learned to engage our senses, cultivate gratitude, minimize distractions, and reflect on our experiences as we savor each bite. We've explored the profound connection between food and well-being, recognizing that what we put on our plates has a profound impact on our health, energy, and vitality. We've also delved into the complexities of emotional eating, offering strategies for identifying and overcoming triggers, as well as practical approaches to managing portion sizes and balancing our meals. We've discovered how to make healthier choices, both at home and when dining out, and how to navigate social situations with confidence and mindfulness. In our exploration of food allergies, sensitivities, and dietary restrictions, we've gained a deeper understanding of the importance of listening to our bodies and making choices that support our unique needs. We've learned about healthy cooking techniques and discovered nutrient-packed recipes that can delight our taste buds and nourish our bodies. Furthermore, we've explored the broader impact of our food choices on the environment and local communities, emphasizing the value of supporting sustainable and ethical food systems. We've also delved into the significance of reducing food waste and adopting a long-term approach to wellness, recognizing that true well-being is a lifelong journey. Throughout this journey, we've encountered setbacks and challenges, but we've also discovered the resilience within ourselves to overcome them. We've embraced self-compassion and cultivated a deeper sense of self-love and self-care. We've learned that the journey to a healthier and more mindful relationship with food is not without its obstacles, but it is a journey worth taking. As we conclude this book, remember that the journey doesn't end here. It continues in the choices you make at every meal, in the moments of mindfulness you bring to your plate, and in the self-compassion and self-love you extend to yourself. "FOOD RELATIONSHIP - A Love Affair with Wellness" is not just a book; it's a guide, a companion, and an invitation to embark on a lifelong love affair with food—one that nourishes your body, mind, and soul. So, as you move forward on your journey, may you savor each bite, practice gratitude, and embrace patience and self-compassion. May you continue to engage your senses, reflect on your experiences, and make choices that align with your well-being. And may you find joy, fulfillment, and a deeper connection with yourself and the world around you through the profound and transformative practice of mindful and balanced eating.